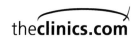

THORACIC SURGERY CLINICS

Thoracic Trauma

GUEST EDITOR
Stephen R. Hazelrigg, MD

CONSULTING EDITOR
Mark K. Ferguson, MD

February 2007 • Volume 17 • Number 1

SAUNDERS

An Imprint of Elsevier, Inc.
PHILADELPHIA LONDON TORONTO MONTREAL SYDNEY TOKYO

W.B. SAUNDERS COMPANY
A Division of Elsevier Inc.

1600 John F. Kennedy Boulevard, Suite 1800 • Philadelphia, Pennsylvania 19103-2899

http://www.theclinics.com

THORACIC SURGERY CLINICS
February 2007
Editor: Catherine Bewick

Volume 17, Number 1
ISSN 1547-4127
ISBN 1-4160-4386-1
978-1-4160-4386-7

The ideas and opinions expressed in *Thoracic Surgery Clinics* do not necessarily reflect those of the Publisher. The Publisher does not assume any responsibility for any injury and/or damage to persons or property arising out of or related to any use of the material contained in this periodical. The reader is advised to check the appropriate medical literature and the product information currently provided by the manufacturer of each drug to be administered to verify the dosage, the method and duration of ad-ministration, or contraindications. It is the responsibility of the treating physician or other health care professional, relying on independent experience and knowledge of the patient, to determine drug do-sages and the best treatment for the patient. Mention of any product in this issue should not be con-strued as endorsement by the contributors, editors, or the Publisher of the product or manufacturers' claims.

Thoracic Surgery Clinics (ISSN 1547-4127) is published quarterly by Elsevier Inc., 360 Park Avenue South, New York, NY 10010-1710. Months of publication are February, May, August, and November. Business and editorial offices: 1600 John F. Kennedy Boulevard, Suite 1800, Philadelphia, PA 19103-2899. Cus-tomer service office: 6277 Sea Harbor Drive, Orlando, FL 32887-4800. Periodicals postage paid at New York, NY, and additional mailing offices. Subscription prices are $198.00 per year (US individuals), $292.00 per year (US institutions), $99.00 per year (US students), $253.00 per year (Canadian indivi-duals), $362.00 per year (Canadian institutions), $127.00 per year (Canadian and foreign students), $253.00 per year (foreign individuals), and $362.00 per year (foreign institutions). Foreign air speed de-livery is included in all *Clinics'* subscription prices. All prices are subject to change without notice. POSTMASTER: Send address changes to *Thoracic Surgery Clinics*, Elsevier Periodicals Customer Service, 6277 Sea Harbor Drive, Orlando, FL 32887-4800. **Customer Service: 1-800-654-2452 (US). From outside of the US, call 1-407-345-4000.** E-mail: hhspcs@wbsaunders.com.

Reprints. For copies of 100 or more, of articles in this publication, please contact Commercial Rights De-partment, Elsevier Inc., 360 Park Avenue South, New York, NY 10010-1710. Tel: (212) 633-3813; Fax: (212) 462-1935; e-mail: reprints@elsevier.com.

Thoracic Surgery Clinics is covered in *Index Medicus* and *EMBASE/Excerpta Medica*.

Printed in the United States of America.

CONSULTING EDITOR

MARK K. FERGUSON, MD, Professor of Surgery, Section of Cardiac and Thoracic Surgery, The University of Chicago, Chicago, Illinois

GUEST EDITOR

STEPHEN R. HAZELRIGG, MD, Professor and Chief, Division of Cardiothoracic Surgery, Department of Surgery, Southern Illinois University School of Medicine, Springfield, Illinois

CONTRIBUTORS

JOSEPH E. BAVARIA, MD, Vice Chair and Professor of Surgery, Division of Cardiovascular Surgery, Hospital of the University of Pennsylvania, Philadelphia, Pennsylvania

WILLIAM T. BRINKMAN, MD, Division of Cardiovascular Surgery, Hospital of the University of Pennsylvania, Philadelphia, Pennsylvania

AYESHA S. BRYANT, MSPH, MD, Assistant Professor, Department of Epidemiology, University of Alabama at Birmingham, Birmingham, Alabama

JOHN B. CALHOON, MD, Professor and Chairman, Division of Cardiothoracic Surgery, Department of Surgery, University of Texas Health Science Center, San Antonio, Texas

ROBERT J. CERFOLIO, MD, Professor of Surgery and Chief, Section of Thoracic Surgery, University of Alabama at Birmingham, Birmingham, Alabama

IBRAHIM B. CETINDAG, MD, Resident, Department of Surgery, Southern Illinois University School of Medicine, Springfield, Illinois

RICHARD EMBREY, MD, Associate Professor, Department of Surgery, Southern Illinois University School of Medicine, Springfield, Illinois

THOMAS GLEASON, MD, Center for Thoracic Aortic Disease, Heart, Lung, and Esophageal Surgery Institute, Cardiothoracic Surgery, University of Pittsburgh Medical Center, Pittsburgh, Pennsylvania

STEPHEN R. HAZELRIGG, MD, Professor and Chief, Division of Cardiothoracic Surgery, Department of Surgery, Southern Illinois University School of Medicine, Springfield, Illinois

SCOTT B. JOHNSON, MD, Associate Professor and Head, Section of General Thoracic Surgery, Division of Cardiothoracic Surgery, Department of Surgery, University of Texas Health Science Center, San Antonio, Texas

RIYAD KARMY-JONES, MD, Heart and Vascular Center, Divisions of Cardiac, Vascular, and Thoracic Surgery, Southwest Washington Medical Center, SWMC Physicians Pavilion, Vancouver, Washington

SANDEEP J. KHANDHAR, MD, Fellow, Minimally Invasive Thoracic Surgery, Division of Cardiothoracic Surgery, Department of Surgery, Duke University Medical Center, Durham, North Carolina

RODNEY J. LANDRENEAU, MD, Professor of Surgery, Heart, Lung, and Esophageal Surgery Institute; Director, Comprehensive Lung Cancer Center, University of Pittsburgh Medical Center, Shadyside Medical Center, Pittsburgh, Pennsylvania

JENNINE LARSON, MD, Chief Resident in General Surgery, Department of Surgery, Southern Illinois University School of Medicine, Springfield, Illinois

JAMES A. LUKETICH, MD, Sampson Family Endowed Chair in Thoracic Oncology and Chief, Heart, Lung, and Esophageal Surgery Institute; Co-Director, Minimally Invasive Surgery Center; Co-Director, Lung Cancer Center; and Director of Thoracic Surgical Oncology, University of Pittsburgh Medical Center, Shadyside Medical Center, Pittsburgh, Pennsylvania

KAMAL A. MANSOUR, MD, Professor of Surgery, Emory University School of Medicine, Atlanta, Georgia

DAN M. MEYER, MD, Sarah M. and Charles E. Seay Distinguished Chair in Thoracic Surgery, Department of Thoracic and Cardiovascular Surgery, University of Texas Southwestern Medical Center at Dallas, Dallas, Texas

DANIEL L. MILLER, MD, Chief, Section of General Thoracic Surgery, Department of Surgery, Emory University and The Emory Clinic, Atlanta, Georgia

KEITH S. NAUNHEIM, MD, The Vallee L. and Melba Willman Professor and Chief of Cardiothoracic Surgery, St. Louis University Medical Center, St. Louis, Missouri

TODD NEIDEEN, MD, Resident, Department of Surgery, Medical College of Wisconsin, Milwaukee, Wisconsin

STEPHEN NICHOLLS, MD, Heart and Vascular Center, Divisions of Cardiac, Vascular, and Thoracic Surgery, Southwest Washington Medical Center, SWMC Physicians Pavilion, Vancouver, Washington

BRIAN L. PETTIFORD, MD, Clinical Assistant Professor, Heart, Lung, and Esophageal Surgery Institute, University of Pittsburgh Medical Center, Shadyside Medical Center, Pittsburgh, Pennsylvania

JAMES R. SCHARFF, MD, Resident in Cardiothoracic Surgery, St. Louis University Medical Center, St. Louis Missouri

JOHN P. SUTYAK, EdM, MD, Associate Professor of Surgery, Department of Surgery; and Director, Southern Illinois Trauma Center, Southern Illinois University School of Medicine, Springfield, Illinois

WILSON Y. SZETO, MD, Division of Cardiovascular Surgery, Hospital of the University of Pennsylvania, Philadelphia, Pennsylvania

CHRISTOPHER D. WOHLTMANN, MD, Assistant Professor of Surgery, Department of Surgery; and Associate Director, Southern Illinois Trauma Center, Southern Illinois University School of Medicine, Springfield, Illinois

DOUGLAS E. WOOD, MD, Professor and Chief of General Thoracic Surgery, and Endowed Chair in Lung Cancer Research, Division of Cardiothoracic Surgery, University of Washington Medical Center, Seattle, Washington

CONTRIBUTORS

CONTENTS

The treatment of thoracic trauma continues to evolve over the years. Initial care of these patients is straightforward and often performed adequately by emergency room physicians and general surgeons. Tertiary care of these patients is multidisciplinary in nature, however, and communication with the thoracic surgeon is essential to minimize mortality and long-term morbidity. Improvement in the understanding of the underlying molecular physiologic mechanisms involved in the various traumatic pathologic processes, and the advancement of diagnostic techniques, minimally invasive approaches, and pharmacologic therapy, all continue to contribute to decreasing the morbidity and mortality of these critically injured patients.

Many victims of thoracic trauma require ICU care and mechanical ventilatory support. Pressure and volume-limited modes assist in the prevention of ventilator-associated lung injury. Ventilator-associated pneumonia is a significant cause of posttraumatic morbidity and mortality. Minimizing ventilator days, secretion control, early nutritional support, and patient positioning are methods to reduce the risk of pneumonia.

Flail chest is an uncommon consequence of blunt trauma. It usually occurs in the setting of a high-speed motor vehicle crash and can carry a high morbidity and mortality. The outcome of flail chest injury is a function of associated injuries. Isolated flail chest may be successfully managed with aggressive pulmonary toilet including facemask oxygen, continuous positive airway pressure, and chest physiotherapy. Surgical stabilization is associated with a faster ventilator wean, shorter ICU time, less hospital cost, and recovery of pulmonary function in a select group of patients with flail chest. There is no role for stabilization for patients who have severe pulmonary contusion. Supportive therapy and pneumatic stabilization is the recommended approach for this patient subset.

Video-Assisted Thoracic Surgical Applications in Thoracic Trauma   73
Ibrahim B. Cetindag, Todd Neideen, and Stephen R. Hazelrigg

> Video-assisted thoracic surgery (VATS) has been used in thoracic trauma for treatment of retained hemothorax, persistent pneumothorax, the diagnosis of diaphragmatic injuries after penetrating trauma, posttraumatic empyema, management of ongoing bleeding, retrieval of foreign bodies, and for traumatic chylothoraces. In some instances VATS has proved more effective than conservative treatment or chest tube placement. Thoracoscopy has proved to have a high degree of sensitivity and specificity in detecting diaphragmatic injuries. The main contraindication to VATS in trauma is patients who require emergency treatment because of hemodynamic instability; in these patients a thoracotomy or sternotomy should be used.

Traumatic Diaphragmatic Injuries   81
James R. Schaff and Keith S. Naunheim

> The best tool to guide the clinician toward the appropriate diagnosis of traumatic diaphragmatic hernia is a high index of suspicion in patients with blunt or appropriate penetrating trauma. Although laparoscopic or thoracoscopic management of such patients may become prevalent with increasing experience, at present the open approach and simple repair remain the mainstays of management. The patient's survival still depends more on the severity of concomitant nondiaphragmatic injuries and in many cases the diaphragmatic laceration is the least worrisome and least morbid of the patient's injuries. Operative repair results in a good outcome in most patients in the absence of other serious injuries.

Cardiac Trauma   87
Richard Embry

> Fifty years ago, nearly all significant cardiac injuries were fatal, many were untreatable, and most undiagnosed until the autopsy suite. In the last 20 years, however, dramatic improvements in prehospital trauma management, new diagnostic modalities, and the availability of cardiac surgery in many hospitals have rendered treatable most cardiac injuries. Knowledge of various types of cardiac injuries, the methods available to facilitate rapid diagnosis, and familiarity with techniques for surgical repair are no longer an academic exercise but a life-saving necessity.

Overview of Great Vessel Trauma   95
William T. Brinkman, Wilson Y. Szeto, and Joseph E. Bavaria

> Traumatic injury to the aorta and the brachiocephalic branches are potentially lethal injuries. Specialized preoperative imaging and medical management can lead to better outcomes in this group of patients. In addition, improved surgical techniques for spinal cord protection have led to decreased morbidity in surgical candidates. Thoracic endovascular stent grafts remain a promising technique; however, long-term data currently are not available.

Endovascular repair of the traumatically injured thoracic aorta has emerged as an exceptionally promising modality that is typically quicker than open repair, with a reduced risk of paralysis. There is a specific set of anatomic criteria that need to be applied, which can be rapidly assessed by the CT angiogram. The enthusiasm for endovascular repair must be tempered by recognition of the complications and lack of long-term follow-up, particularly in younger patients. Surgeons who are skilled in open aortic repair must not only be involved, but should take on a leadership role during the planning, deployment, and follow-up of these patients. As more specific devices become available, and more follow-up is accrued, the role of endovascular stents will continue to grow.

FORTHCOMING ISSUES

ELSEVIER
SAUNDERS

Thorac Surg Clin 17 (2007) xi

THORACIC
SURGERY
CLINICS

Preface

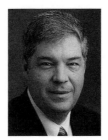

Stephen R. Hazelrigg, MD
Guest Editor

It has been a real pleasure for me to assist in organizing experts to contribute to the topic of thoracic trauma that is covered in this issue of the *Thoracic Surgery Clinics*. My goal from the outset was to provide a comprehensive issue to cover the pertinent areas in thoracic trauma. Although most of us participate, at least peripherally, in the management of trauma patients, only a few of us really spend a majority of our time in this area. Hence, an issue like this can prove to be a very valuable resource.

Some of the topics that are covered in this issue—such as endovascular management for vascular injuries—are particularly timely. Thoracic vascular trauma has traditionally been managed by thoracic surgeons. We best understand the disease process and management options; however, the endovascular techniques threaten to change that relationship. Clearly, if we do not learn these skills

we will be relinquishing our primary role in thoracic vascular trauma.

In the end, I am very pleased with the content of this issue, and I hope that the readership will feel the same way. I wish to conclude by thanking the contributing authors for their time and effort in summarizing this area of thoracic surgery. I think they have done an outstanding job.

Stephen R. Hazelrigg, MD
Division of Cardiothoracic Surgery
Department of Surgery
Southern Illinois University School of Medicine
800 N. Rutledge, Room D319
P.O. Box 19638
Springfield, IL 62794-9638, USA

E-mail address: shazelrigg@siumed.edu

ELSEVIER
SAUNDERS

Thorac Surg Clin 17 (2007) 1–9

THORACIC
SURGERY
CLINICS

Overview of Thoracic Trauma in the United States

Sandeep J. Khandhar, MD[a],*, Scott B. Johnson, MD[b],
John H. Calhoon, MD[b]

[a]Division of Cardiothoracic Surgery, Department of Surgery, Duke University Medical Center,
Durham, NC 27710, USA
[b]Division of Cardiothoracic Surgery, Department of Surgery, University of Texas Health Science Center,
7703 Floyd Curl Drive, Mail Code 7841, San Antonio, TX 78229, USA

Historical perspective

The treatment of thoracic trauma has undergone tremendous evolution. Despite substantial progress, the death toll from these injuries remains high. The history of thoracic trauma is documented as early as 1600 BC in the Edwin Smith Surgical Papyrus written in ancient Egypt, probably by Imhotep, builder of the Great Pyramid [1]. He describes 48 cases of trauma, four of which involved the chest. One case describes flail chest with bony crepitation and injuries to the overlying soft tissues. The author believed that the condition was hopeless and recommended no treatment [2,3]. In the 400s BC, Hippocrates described hemoptysis after rib fracture, but notably recognized that the hemoptysis signified injury to the underlying lung and was much more serious than a simple rib fracture [3]. He firmly wrapped the chest with linen to stabilize the fractured ribs for a period of 20 days, unless there was hemoptysis, in which case the therapy continued for 40 days [4]. The stabilization of the chest with binding dressings, a practice now abandoned, would continue well into the twentieth century. Aristotle, despite his forward thinking in the mid 300s BC, stated: "The heart alone of all the viscera cannot withstand serious injury. This is to be expected because when the main source of strength (the heart) is destroyed there is no aid that can be brought to the other organs which depend on

it." In the 100s BC, Galen noted that when wounds of the heart were seen in gladiators, they were uniformly fatal [5]. Early accounts of thoracic trauma in these literary works of art clearly document the appreciation for the vitality of the chest and reflect the mysticism with which the organs of the chest were held.

In the eighteenth century, Laurence Heister described the adherence of the lung to the parietal pleura in empyema and the prudence of inserting a finger into the pleural space to gently displace the lung before inserting the trochar used for drainage of the "peccant humors." In 1773, William Bromfield performed the first thoracentesis for traumatic pneumothorax and accurately described the pathophysiology of tension pneumothorax [4]. Johns Jones [6] wrote the first book on surgery in the United States in 1776 and spoke of traumatic pneumothorax and its treatment. This book, *Plain, Concise, Practical Remarks on the Treatment of Wounds and Fractures*, became the manual for surgeons during the Revolutionary War. Jones was also the friend and physician to both Benjamin Franklin and George Washington. The concept of aspirating air in the treatment of pneumothorax, of which Jones wrote, was quickly and thoroughly condemned by John Bell, a Scottish anatomist and surgeon, who proposed in 1795 that re-expansion of the lung would cause an underlying lung injury to bleed. This mistaken fear and condemnation continued until World War II [4].

The modern art of physical diagnosis was initiated by Laennec [7] in 1819 when he described the auscultation of the chest with his monumental

* Corresponding author.
  E-mail address: sandeep.khandhar@duke.edu
(S.J. Khandhar).

1547-4127/07/$ - see front matter © 2007 Elsevier Inc. All rights reserved.
doi:10.1016/j.thorsurg.2007.02.004

invention, the stethoscope. The first use of the term "pulmonary contusion" was by surgeon Guillaume Dupuytren in a posthumous publication in 1839. The abandonment of thoracentesis in the treatment of pneumothorax was largely secondary to the development of empyema, because the antiseptic technique had not yet been introduced. Dupuytren is credited with performing 50 thoracenteses with 48 deaths. When he developed empyema, he refused thoracentesis, stating that he "would rather die by the hand of God than by that of surgeons." The introduction of anesthesia and asepsis occurred in the latter half of the nineteenth century. The first English textbook devoted exclusively to thoracic surgery was written in 1896 by London surgeon, Stephen Paget. A full chapter in this book focused on nonpenetrating chest trauma and furthered the development of the pathophysiologic basis for chest trauma. He stated: "As a rule, any deep laceration in simple fracture of the ribs is due to the violence that broke the ribs, not to the actual entry of the sharp fragments into the lung" [4].

The first successful repair of a cardiac wound came on September 9, 1896, by Ludwig Rehn of Frankfurt, Germany. This event marked the beginning of cardiac surgery [5]. The first successful thoracotomy for a lacerated lung was performed by the German surgeon Kofstein in 1898. The discovery of x-rays in 1895 by Roentgen launched the technologic advances seen in the twentieth century [4].

Over the last hundred years, most of what has been learned has been gleaned from war time. In World War I, chest injuries were the cause of 37% of battlefield deaths. The probability of succumbing to a penetrating wound of the chest was 74% [8,9]. Experience with penetrating chest trauma during World War I was dominated by sepsis of the chest wall and pleural space. One fourth of all hemothoraces became infected and half of these died. By the end of World War I, positive airway pressure anesthesia, blood transfusion, and a clearer understanding of cardiopulmonary physiology all helped pave the way for modern era treatment of otherwise fatal injuries. Chest injuries were the cause of 34% of battlefield deaths during World War II. The probability of succumbing to a penetrating wound of the chest was 61%. When one totals all forms of thoracic wounds, both blunt and penetrating, the case fatality rate for a soldier who sustained a thoracic injury decreased from 24% to 8% from World War I to World War II [8]. The importance of

tracheal suctioning and pulmonary toilet, technical advances in suture material, pioneering techniques making anatomic pulmonary resection a possibility, and the introduction of antimicrobial agents (sulfonamides followed by penicillin) were all considered clinical advances made during World War II [9]. These advances, coupled with the Industrial Revolution, set the stage for the current understanding and management of thoracic trauma.

Epidemiology

The death toll from traumatic thoracic injuries has largely stabilized and their resultant morbidity is decreasing as understanding of the disease process improves. It has been well established that 25% of traumatic deaths are secondary to injuries to the thorax. In motor vehicle crashes, 45% to 50% of unrestrained drivers have a thoracic injury and 25% of all motor vehicle driver deaths are known to have a thoracic injury. In patients presenting with penetrating trauma, 40% have a thoracic injury, whereas with blunt trauma, 33% have a thoracic injury [10,11]. A transected aorta is thought to be the cause of death in approximately 12% to 30% of patients who die at the scene from blunt trauma [12].

In 2003, accidents (unintentional injuries) ranked fifth overall in total number of deaths (109,277) in the United States behind diseases of the heart (685,089); malignant neoplasms (556,902); cerebrovascular diseases (157,689); and chronic lower respiratory diseases (126,382). Grouping all injury-related deaths (to include suicide, homicide, undetermined, and war-related deaths, in addition to accidents), the total number was 164,002, making injury-related deaths the third most common cause for death in the United States. This makes the traumatic death rate 56.4 per 100,000 people, or 6.7% of the percentage of all deaths [13]. This death rate has slowly risen over the previous 4 years, with the low occurring in the year 2000, at 52.7 per 100,000 [14]. Motor vehicle–related injuries, firearms, stabbings, other assaults, and falls account for more than half of these deaths (58.1%). The male/female ratio for firearm-related deaths is 6.5:1 [13].

Pathophysiology

General concepts

Thoracic injuries leave little room for error in their diagnosis and management. If improperly managed they are frequently fatal, whereas massive insults can usually be treated by simple maneuvers with generally excellent results [15]. The understanding of pathophysiologic processes and the mechanisms of traumatic injury is crucial in the management of these patients. The thorax is the only area of the body where five separate mechanisms for early loss of life coexist [11]:

1. Airway obstruction from tracheobronchial injuries, pulmonary secretions, or hemorrhage
2. Loss of oxygenation and ventilation capability from pneumothorax, hemothorax, or pulmonary contusion
3. Exsanguination
4. Cardiac failure from cardiac contusion or valve rupture
5. Cardiac tamponade

The ability to understand these injuries better has not only reduced the mortality attributable to these injuries, but has also significantly reduced morbidity. Industrial advances, such as the advent of CT scanning, MRI, and thoracoscopy, has enabled the thoracic surgeon to better understand and diagnose patients who have sustained significant thoracic trauma.

Blunt versus penetrating injury

Trauma has been divided broadly into two main categories for ease of discussion: blunt and penetrating [16]. This differentiation is important with regard to multisystem management. Because of the higher likelihood of multisystem injury in blunt trauma, its morbidity and mortality is consequently higher. Motor vehicle crashes remain the number one cause of blunt chest trauma despite the improvements in vehicle design, airbags, and the use of seatbelts [17]. Gunshot and stab wounds account for the majority of penetrating injuries. In 2004 alone, motor vehicle accidents resulted in 43,947 deaths and firearm injuries resulted in 29,036 deaths.

Ballistics

It is important to have a basic understanding of wound ballistics and the wounding power of missiles to understand better the mechanism of injury caused by these forces [18]. The destruction of tissue on impact is directly proportional to the absorbed kinetic energy (KE), which is derived from the formula $KE = \frac{1}{2} M(V_1-V_2)^2$, where M represents the weight of the projectile (defined as mass divided by the gravity constant), V_1 represents the striking velocity, and V_2 represents the exit velocity [3,8,18–20]. In ballistics, a distinction is made between low- and high-velocity missiles, with a velocity of more than 2500 ft/s being designated high velocity. This in general corresponds to a KE greater than 750 ft-lb. Lower KE missiles tend to have similar-sized entrance and exit wounds and cause damage primarily to the structures that are in the missile's path. Higher KE missiles are more prone to cavitation, causing significant injury to tissues surrounding the path of the missile. Bullets that shatter or tumble have a slower exit velocity and impart more energy to the affected tissues, thereby resulting in more cavitation [19]. Cavitation is defined as a momentary acceleration of tissue in all directions away from the tract of a missile, producing a cavity of subatmospheric pressure. This cavity collapses because of the resultant vacuum effect, then reforms and collapses several times with diminishing amplitude until all motion ceases. This "shockwave" that results from the dispersement of this rebounding energy acts as the source of injury to surrounding structures. These missiles result in exit wounds that are substantially larger than their corresponding entrance wounds. In addition, the cavitation results in nerve damage, thrombosis, or rupture of vessels and even fractures of bones within the vicinity of the missile's path, although no direct contact with the missile may occur. Dense organs, such as bone and liver, absorb more energy resulting in more injury. Lungs, which have a much lower density, absorb less energy and fortunately suffer less of an injury [3,20]. This explains the low frequency of operative intervention in penetrating chest trauma. Some typical energy levels delivered by some of the more common weapons seen in civilian trauma are as follows [17]:

.22-caliber handgun = 75 ft-lb
.38-caliber handgun = 350 ft-lb
.357 magnum revolver = 750 ft-lb
Hunting rifle = 1200–3000 ft-lb

The pleural space

The pleural space is a potential space between the visceral and parietal pleura. The accumulation of blood or air within this space is considered pathologic and may result from injury to almost any structure within the thoracic cavity. The accumulation of blood or air within the pleural space may be diagnosed by simple methods including physical examination or by plain radiographic evaluation. Placement of a chest tube usually effectively evacuates the resultant air or blood and is most often the only therapeutic intervention necessary for patients who sustain thoracic trauma [1,11,21–24].

Tension pneumothorax is the result of unevacuated air within the pleural space in the setting of an injury to the visceral pleura that continues to fill the space on inspiration without a route for egress, because the defect in the visceral pleura functionally acts as a one-way valve [25]. The intrapleural pressure rises and mediastinal structures begin to shift away from the injured hemithorax, resulting in diminished venous return as the superior vena cava and inferior vena cava begin to occlude resulting in fatal hypotension. This is a clinical diagnosis and should be aggressively treated even before obtaining the usual radiographic confirmation.

A hemothorax may occur from injury to the (1) pulmonary parenchyma, (2) hilar vessels, (3) heart with a communicating defect in the pericardium and pleura, (4) great vessels with an opening in the pleura, (5) intercostal vessels, or (6) internal thoracic arteries. Lung parenchymal bleeding usually ceases spontaneously as a result of the low pressure in the pulmonary vessels, the compressive effect of the shed blood in a closed space, and a high concentration of thromboplastin in the lung [3]. Bleeding from any of the major vessels or an intercostal artery or from the internal thoracic arteries, however, may require prompt operative intervention [15]. The natural history of a large, undrained hemothorax consists of clotting of the blood followed by fibroblast proliferation at the periphery of the clotted hemothorax as early as the seventh day postinjury. Over the next several weeks, mature fibrous tissue encases the clot forming a peel, which is loosely adherent to both the visceral and parietal pleural surfaces. This peel continues to increase in firmness, thickness, and adhesiveness to the pleura over time and can cause a significant restrictive defect (fibrothorax) in the adjacent lung if left untreated [15,26]. Another prominent mechanism at play is that of blood cell lysis leading to an increased osmotic load and large serosanguinous pleural effusion, which develops from a relatively small amount of retained blood over a few days (Trinkle, personal communication, 1981). Alternatively, a retained hemothorax may become secondarily infected. This may present in delayed fashion as an

empyema and require extensive surgical debridement or resection.

The issue of extra-anatomic air arises frequently in the management of thoracic trauma patients. Extra-anatomic air present within the thorax generally takes the form of subcutaneous air, pneumomediastinum, or pneumopericardium. Each of these entities represents a pathologic process whose clinical significance is largely variable. The mechanisms by which the introduction of extra-anatomic air into the thoracic cavity can occur include the following [26]:

1. Perforation of the trachea, bronchial tree, or esophagus
2. Injury of the lung
3. Injury of the face, which tracts through the fascial planes into the neck
4. Injury to the retroperitoneal space, which tracts through the diaphragmatic hiatus
5. Introduced from the outside as a result of a penetrating injury

Indications for thoracotomy

The indications for thoracotomy for both blunt and penetrating trauma are based on physical findings, radiographic and echocardiographic imaging, and most importantly the clinical course of the patient. The following represent most of the 15% to 30% of thoracic injuries that require operative intervention [1,11,21–24]:

1. Acute hemodynamic deterioration with cardiac arrest in the trauma center
2. Cardiac tamponade
3. Vascular injury at the thoracic outlet or great vessels
4. Massive airleak from a chest tube
5. Tracheal or bronchial injury
6. Esophageal injury
7. Retained hemothorax or its sequelae
8. Traumatic diaphragmatic hernia
9. Traumatic cardiac valvular or aneurysmal lesions
10. Traumatic thoracic pseudoaneurysms or aortic disruption
11. Tracheoesophageal fistula

The chest wall

The chest wall represents the first line of defense against both blunt and penetrating injury to the chest. Protection is rendered largely from the ribs, clavicles, scapula, and sternum. Rib fractures are the most common injury seen in blunt trauma victims but are less likely to be seen in children secondary to the (greenstick) rib's increased compliance. Rib fractures can result in significant chest wall discomfort. This pain typically limits chest wall excursion and increases the propensity for hypoventilation, atelectasis, and eventually pneumonia, especially in the setting of an underlying pulmonary contusion. Elderly patients and those with poor pulmonary reserve are at the highest risk [27].

Although chest wall immobilization may reduce pain, which was historically and traditionally the focus of treatment in these injuries, immobilization of the chest wall impairs pulmonary toilet and increases the risk of atelectasis, compromised gas exchange, and eventually pneumonia to occur. The mainstay of treatment is pain control (narcotics, if necessary), along with good pulmonary toilet.

Sternal fractures can be associated with underlying myocardial contusions, which can be manifested as dysrhythmias and should warrant telemetry monitoring. Clavicle fractures can be painful but only occasionally result in major vascular or neurologic injury. Scapular fractures and first rib fractures are markers of significant force and can be a marker for other, more life-threatening injuries that should be sought after carefully [27]. In one series of 52 patients with scapular fractures, most (42) sustained other injuries [28]. In another series of 55 patients, the mortality in patients with a first rib fracture was 36%, with the predominant cause of death being an associated intracranial injury [29].

A large chest wall defect can result in a sucking chest wound or large open pneumothorax. This phenomenon occurs when the injury consists of a large chest wall defect in addition to a sizable visceral pleural injury. A tension pneumothorax usually does not occur because there is a large chest wall defect to allow egress of air unless the wound is covered in an occlusive fashion. Hypoxia and respiratory acidosis caused by hypoventilation and often asphyxiation can result if left untreated. Normally, inspiration of air occurs when the chest wall expands, resulting in a negative intrapleural pressure. This negative pressure then draws air into the lungs allowing them to fill. With a sucking chest wound, any negative pressure that is generated on the ipsilateral side instead results in air entering the wound at atmospheric pressure (rather than through the trachea), which then is unavailable for gas exchange at the alveolar-capillary level. As the size of the defect increases, air preferentially enters the wound rather than the trachea [25]. Although some air is drawn to the normal contralateral side, this functionally represents the ventilation of one lung with the perfusion of both. Treatment is the coverage of the defect to prevent air entry along with immediate placement of a chest tube to prevent the development of a tension pneumothorax and to facilitate more normal pulmonary ventilation.

Flail chest is another injury of the chest wall that occurs when more than two ribs are broken in two or more places resulting in a free floating segment of the chest wall. This was originally thought pathologic, because there would be paradoxical motion of this segment during the respiratory cycle causing recirculation of air from the affected lung into the contralateral lung during inspiration and from the contralateral lung into the affected lung during exhalation. This concept was the so-called theory of "Pendelluft" [19,30]. Therapeutic efforts were directed at stabilization of the chest wall [27]. In reality, morbidity of this injury is probably related more primarily to the underlying pulmonary contusion. Mainstays of flail chest treatment are directed at limiting the underlying pulmonary contusion by judicious fluid resuscitation and the use of diuretics as tolerated in conjunction with pain control to facilitate and maintain good ventilation and pulmonary toilet. They were popularized by Trinkle and colleagues in the 1970s. Mechanical ventilation may be required; internal fixation is rarely required but may be useful in some cases.

Pulmonary parenchyma

Injuries of the visceral pleura can result from blunt or penetrating trauma. The severity of a penetrating injury is directly related to the depth of penetration, the kinetic energy dissipated to the tissues, and its proximity to the hilum. Blunt injury can also result in significant injuries to the pulmonary parenchyma and pleura. A pneumothorax, pneumomediastinum, or subcutaneous emphysema can result and usually be adequately treated with a simple chest tube. High-energy missiles and severe blunt trauma can result in the development of large ventilation-perfusion defects. Injuries of this magnitude can trigger the inflammatory cascade resulting in significant neutrophilic infiltration, hypervascularity, capillary leak, and edema. This concept was introduced in the 1940s macroscopically as "traumatic wet-lung syndrome"; however, the complex microvascular understanding of the inflammatory response did not develop until recently [15,25]. Despite the increase in overall blood flow to the area as a result of this inflammatory process, gas exchange is severely impaired as the alveolus fills with fluid and the alveolar-capillary membrane becomes infiltrated limiting the diffusion of oxygen and carbon dioxide. Three mechanisms have been proposed as etiologic factors for this complex injury [3,31]:

1. An explosive effect from the overexpansion of intrapulmonary air secondary to a positive-pressure concussive wave resulting in stretching and rupture of alveoli
2. An inertial effect as a result of deceleration where low-density alveoli are stripped away from heavier bronchial structures
3. The Spauling effect, in which a concussive wave encounters a liquid-gas interface, such as the alveolar wall with the intra-alveolar gas, and causes a disruption of the interface

If the process is severe and localized, lung necrosis may result requiring resection. Usually, the process is diffuse as a result of (1) increased mucous production, (2) blood and edema fluid that fill the bronchial tree, (3) decreased surfactant concentrations, and (4) increased capillary permeability. These processes not only affect the directly injured portions of the lung but also the adjacent uninjured lung [3]. Treatment is generally supportive. Pain control [32] is crucial to prevent the infectious complications of compromised pulmonary toilet, atelectasis, and stasis. Coughing should be encouraged, particularly in the elderly, and tracheal aspiration by catheter, bronchoscopy, or even tracheostomy may become necessary [15]. Intravenous fluid administration should be restricted to avoid adding to the transudative insult. Mechanical ventilation may be necessary, especially if the condition degenerates to the clinical picture of acute respiratory distress syndrome.

The major airways

A major tracheobronchial injury should be suspected if there are large amounts of air within the subcutaneous space, mediastinum, or pleural space. In addition, if the pleural space has been injured and there is a large, persistent air leak

from a chest tube or failure of the lung to expand properly, a tracheobronchial injury should be suspected [26]. Occasionally, in the setting of a completely transected bronchus, the injured area may be sealed off by clot or fibrin deposition and an air leak may not be present. In this case, the affected lung is collapsed and not ventilated, resulting in a delayed diagnosis. This may lead to chronic atelectasis and volume loss or a suppurative, infected process. There are three mechanisms that help explain these injuries in blunt force trauma [33]:

1. Anterior-posterior compression of the chest resulting in the widening of the carina and shearing off of the right mainstem bronchus.
2. Sudden increase in intrathoracic pressure against a closed glottis resulting in a blowout of the membranous portion of the largest bronchi. This is where the wall tension is highest according to the Law of Laplace, and the most likely area of rupture.
3. A rapid deceleration injury can cause a transverse laceration in the trachea between its two points of fixation, namely near the cricoid cartilage and usually within 2 cm of the carina.

Smaller airway injuries generally heal with time and can be definitively treated with tube thoracostomy alone; however, tracheal, mainstem bronchial, or lobar bronchial injuries usually require operative repair or parenchymal resection.

The great vessels

Aortic injuries are the most common of the great vessel injuries and the most lethal. There are three primary locations that intimal tears or transections occur from blunt force trauma: (1) near the ligamentum arteriosum, (2) at the aortic root, and (3) at the diaphragm. These areas represent points of fixation and are prone to shear stress during a rapid change in bodily velocity. The tears that occur are usually transverse and usually involve both the intima and media. If the surrounding adventitia is unable to contain the rupture, fatal exsanguination inevitably occurs. If the patient is fortunate enough to survive the initial insult, the pseudoaneurysm that results is contained only by the adventitia and surrounding mediastinal and pleural surfaces [25]. Initial medical treatment of these patients should be aimed at decreasing the aortic wall stress before definitive repair using drugs that reduce heart rate, mean arterial pressure, and afterload. Timing of surgical repair may be safely delayed in certain situations if associated injuries are present that preclude heparinization or single lung ventilation, or if other significant co-morbid conditions are present. Thoracic endograft-ing is a new technique that may play a role in the management of these complex injuries.

Subclavian injuries occur largely secondary to penetrating trauma and can pose an operative challenge with regard to exposure and obtaining both proximal and distal arterial control, given the much protected location of the subclavian artery. It is important to remember that the presence of a distal pulse does not rule out a proximal injury, because an artery can be completely transected with blood flow preserved through the perivascular tissues. In addition, the absence of bleeding or hematoma does not necessarily rule out an intimal flap or complete vascular thrombosis [34].

Penetrating pulmonary injuries are managed with tube thoracostomy alone in most (ie, approximately 75%) patients [1,11,21–24]. Of those who require operative intervention, 24% have been shown to require repair of pulmonary hilar or major parenchymal injuries [24]. Pulmo-nary resections in this setting have been shown to carry a mortality rate of 30% to 60% [24,26,35]. Death typically ensues from exsangui-nating hemorrhage or massive air embolism [26,35,36]. Air embolism occurs in the setting of a fistulous connection between a bronchus and a pulmonary vein. With spontaneous respiration, the pressure differential favors a gradient from the vein to the bronchus resulting in hemoptysis in 22% of these patients. With positive pressure ventilation or with Valsalva-type respiration, the gradient is reversed and results in systemic air embolism. This may present in three ways [19]: (1) focal neurologic defect; (2) sudden cardiovas-cular collapse from embolization to the coronar-ies; and (3) froth in the arterial blood gas sample.

In addition to these acute complications, major pulmonary resections, especially pneumonectomy, can be complicated by postoperative pulmonary hypertension. The initial hypovolemic shock re-sults in a more profound increase in pulmonary vascular resistance as compared with systemic vascular resistance, possibly because of shock-induced thromboxane and neutrophil activity on the pulmonary vascular bed. Coupled with a major pulmonary resection, this can dramatically in-crease right ventricular afterload and lead to right

ventricular failure with deviation of the interven-tricular septum and resultant left ventricular dysfunction. A 20% to 25% incidence of cardiac arrhythmias, usually atrial fibrillation, can further add to the cardiac insult [26].

The esophagus

Injury to the esophagus can rapidly lead to mediastinitis if left untreated [16]. An injury to the cervical esophagus typically drains into the deep cervical fascia, which is in continuity with the me-diastinum. An injury to the proximal two thirds of the esophagus often drains into the right pleural space and results in a right-sided effusion. Con-versely, injury to the distal third of the esophagus typically drains into the left pleural space. Injury to the very distal esophagus may present as free intra-abdominal air, peritonitis, or as a subphrenic abscess if diagnosis is delayed.

Most injuries to the esophagus as a result of penetrating trauma occur in the neck. Patients with thoracic and abdominal esophageal pene-trating injuries often succumb from injuries to adjacent vital structures. Blunt injury to the esophagus is relatively rare, but can result in a rupture of the esophagus from anteroposterior compression against closed upper and lower esophageal sphincters. This usually occurs at the level of the carina where the esophagus may be tethered by subcarinal lymph nodes [27].

Subcutaneous air and pleural effusions are the hallmarks of esophageal injury. As opposed to tracheobronchial injuries, which create a large amount of air in abnormal locations, the resultant air from an esophageal injury can be very subtle and a challenge to diagnose. Mediastinal emphy-sema may be appreciated on physical examination as a "crunch" with each heartbeat, known as Hamman's sign [25]. To increase diagnostic yield, a combination of diagnostic modalities may be necessary. Esophagoscopy in combination with barium swallow results in the highest diagnostic yield. Each method has an individual specificity of 85% to 90%, but approaches 100% when both are used together [26]. Management of these injuries can be difficult but primary repair is pre-ferred when possible, although resection and diversion may be required.

The diaphragm

A small injury to the diaphragm may go undiagnosed initially and present years later as a diaphragmatic hernia. Diaphragmatic hernias classically present in one of three phases [27,37]:

1. Acute phase: Occurs shortly after injury with signs and symptoms related to the intra-thoracic and intra-abdominal structures
2. Interval phase: Symptomatically silent for days to years, during which time there is progressive herniation from the abdomen to the chest because of the differential pressure during the respiratory cycle
3. Late phase: Symptoms occur as a result of complications of herniated viscera, namely intestinal obstruction or gangrene in addition to respiratory or cardiac compression

Diaphragmatic injuries are much more common on the left side because the right side is somewhat protected by the liver. The right side, when injured, is less likely to produce late complications because the defect is often sealed by the liver [27]. Thoracoscopy or laparoscopy can be a useful adjunct in the diagnosis of these injuries.

The heart

Blunt injury to the heart usually manifests as nonspecific EKG changes, elevated enzymes, and most importantly arrhythmias. The myocardial injury results in swelling, which may affect the conduction system. Patients suspected of sustaining a significant cardiac injury should be monitored on telemetry for at least 24 to 48 hours. Less commonly, blunt trauma may result in chamber rupture, usually of the atrium; 80% to 90% of these injuries result in immediate death. Those patients who do survive their initial injury usually present with pericardial tamponade [27]. Occasionally, a blunt injury results in rupture of a papillary muscle, chordae tendineae, or valve leaflet resulting in acute valvular insufficiency. Timing and necessity of repair is predicated on the severity of symptoms [16]. Delayed complications include aneurysm formation and permanent conduction defects [19].

Penetrating injuries to the heart are often fatal. The degree of tamponade or hemorrhage that occurs is related to the size and depth of injury to the heart and the size of the resultant pericardial defect. The pericardium often seals with clot or surrounding fat resulting in control of hemorrhage. It is important to remember that even as little as 60 to 100 mL of blood in the pericardium may produce clinical tamponade [38]. As blood accumulates in the pericardium, stroke volume

decreases and heart rate increases to maintain cardiac output. Deep inspiration lowers intrathoracic pressure, thereby allowing the augmentation of right ventricular diastolic filling. This causes septal shift to the left and a further decrement in left ventricular stroke volume resulting in an exaggerated fall in systolic blood pressure during inspiration known as "pulsus paradoxus." The overall increase in right atrial pressure results in jugular venous distention. The decrease in cardiac output starts the vicious cycle of hypotension, systemic acidosis, and myocardial ischemia, which further reduces cardiac output [38]. Patients who present with pericardial tamponade may be salvaged by pericardiocentesis, pericardial window, or emergency thoracotomy followed by definitive operative repair. Echocardiography has become the mainstay of diagnosis of cardiac injury. Anesthetic management is important to avoid the risk of circulatory collapse during induction caused by vasodilation. In rare patients where any vasodilation could be adverse, a pericardial window done under local anesthesia drains the tamponade partially, allowing for safe complete anesthetic induction and definitive repair. Most wounds of the heart can be repaired using pledgeted sutures on long needles. Lacerations near the coronaries may require horizontal mattress sutures thrown below the coronary to preserve flow. The left anterior descending is the most common coronary injured. Injuries to the distal third of the vessel may be ligated. Injuries to the proximal two thirds should be bypassed.

Summary

Most patients with injuries to the chest ($\sim$75%) can usually be managed expectantly with simple tube thoracostomy and volume resuscitation [1,11,21–24]. As a result, initial care of these patients is usually straightforward and often performed adequately by emergency room physicians and general surgeons. Tertiary care of these patients is often multidisciplinary in nature, however, and communication with the thoracic surgeon is essential to minimize mortality and long-term morbidity. Improvement in the understanding of the underlying molecular physiologic mechanisms involved in the various traumatic pathologic processes, and the advancement of diagnostic techniques, minimally invasive approaches, and pharmacologic therapy, all continue to contribute to decreasing the morbidity and mortality of these critically injured patients.

References

[1] Wall MJ Jr, Huh J, Mattox KL. Thoracotomy. In: Moore EE, Feliciano DV, Mattox KL, editors. Trauma. 5th edition. New York: The McGraw-Hill Companies, Inc.; 2004. p. 493–503.

[2] Breasted JH. The Edwin Smith surgical papyrus, vol. 1. Chicago: University of Chicago Press; 1930.

[3] Boyd AD, Glassman LR. Trauma to the lung. Chest Surg Clin N Am 1997;7(2):263–84.

[4] Wagner RB, Slivko B. Highlights of the history of nonpenetrating chest trauma. Surg Clin North Am 1989;69(1):1–14.

[5] Asensio JA, Stewart BM, Murray J. Penetrating cardiac injuries. Surg Clin North Am 1996;76(4):685–724.

[6] Jones J. Plain concise practical remarks on the treatment of wounds and fractures: to which is added, a short appendix on camp and military hospitals: principally designed for the use of young military and naval surgeons in North-America. Philadelphia: Robert Bell; 1776.

[7] Laennec RTH. A treatise on the diseases of the chest in which they are described according to their diagnosis established on a new principle by means of acoustic instruments. 1st American edition. Philadelphia: J. Webster; 1823.

[8] Beebe GW, DeBakey ME. Battle casualties. Springfield (IL): Charles C. Thomas Publisher, Ltd.; 1952. p. 114–6.

[9] Bellamy RF. History of surgery for penetrating chest trauma. Chest Surg Clin N Am 2000;10(1):55–70.

[10] Lee RB. Traumatic injury of the cervicothoracic trachea and major bronchi. Chest Surg Clin N Am 1997;7(2):285–305.

[11] Feliciano DV. The diagnostic and therapeutic approach to chest trauma. Semin Thorac Cardiovasc Surg 1992;4(3):156–62.

[12] Mattox KL, Wall MJ. Historical review of blunt injury to the thoracic aorta. Chest Surg Clin N Am 2000;10(1):167–82.

[13] Hoyert DL, Heron MP, Murphy SL, et al. Deaths: Final Data for 2003. National Vital Statistics Reports. Vol 54, No 13. Hyattsville (MD): National Center for Health Statistics; 2006. p. 5, 9–10, 78–81.

[14] Miniño AM, Anderson RN, Fingerhut LA, et al. Deaths: Injuries, 2002. National Vital Statistics Reports. Vol 54, No 10. Hyattsville (MD): National Center for Health Statistics; 2006. p. 32–7.

[15] Webb WR. Thoracic trauma. Surg Clin North Am 1974;54(5):1179–92.

[16] Blalock JB, Ochsner JL. Management of thoracic trauma. Surg Clin North Am 1966;46(6):1513–24.

[17] Calhoon JH, Trinkle JK. Pathophysiology of chest trauma. Chest Surg Clin N Am 1997;7(2):199–211.

[18] Rich HM. Missile injuries. Am J Surg 1980;139:414.

[19] Trunkey DD. Torso trauma. Curr Probl Surg 1987;24(4):208–49.

[20] Swan KG, Reiner DS, Blackwood JM. Wound ballistics and principles of management. Mil Med 1987;152:29–34.

[21] Siemens R, Polk HC, Gray LA, et al. Indications for thoracotomy following penetrating thoracic injury. J Trauma 1977;17(7):493–500.

[22] Kish G, Kozloff L, Joseph WL, et al. Indications for early thoracotomy in the management of chest trauma. Ann Thorac Surg 1976;22(1):23–8.

[23] Graham JM, Mattox KL, Beall AC Jr. Penetrating trauma of the lung. J Trauma 1979;19:665–9.

[24] Robinson PD, Harman PK, Trinkle JK, et al. Management of penetrating lung injuries in civilian practice. J Thorac Cardiovasc Surg 1988;95:184–90.

[25] Hughes RK. Thoracic trauma. Ann Thorac Surg 1965;1(6):778–804.

[26] Richardson JD, Miller FB, Carrillo EH, et al. Complex thoracic injuries. Surg Clin North Am 1996;76(4):725–48.

[27] Calhoon JH, Grover FL, Trinkle JK. Chest trauma: approach and management. Clin Chest Med 1992;13(1):55–67.

[28] Imitani RJ. Fractures of the scapula: a review of 53 fractures. J Trauma 1975;15:473–8.

[29] Richardson JD, McElvein RB, Trinkle JK. First rib fracture: a hallmark of severe trauma. Ann Surg 1975;181:251–4.

[30] Maloney JV Jr, Schmutzer KJ, Raschke E. Paradoxical respiration and "Pendelluft". J Thorac Cardiovasc Surg 1961;41:291.

[31] Ratliff JL, Fletcher JR, Kopriva C, et al. Pulmonary contusion: a continuing management problem. J Thorac Cardiovasc Surg 1971;62:638–44.

[32] Fouché Y, Tarantino DP. Anesthetic considerations in chest trauma. Chest Surg Clin N Am 1997;7(2):227–38.

[33] Kirsh MM, Orringer MB, Behrendt DM, et al. Management of tracheobronchial disruption secondary to nonpenetrating trauma. Ann Thorac Surg 1976;22:93–101.

[34] Wall MJ, Granchi T, Liscum K, et al. Penetrating thoracic vascular injuries. Surg Clin North Am 1996;76(4):749–61.

[35] Estrera AS, Pass LJ, Platt MR. Systemic arterial air embolism in penetrating lung injury. Ann Thorac Surg 1990;50:257–61.

[36] Ho AM. Is emergency thoracotomy always the most appropriate immediate intervention for systemic air embolism after lung trauma? Chest 1999;116:234–7.

[37] Arom KV. Diaphragmatic injuries. In: Trinkle JK, Grover FL, editors. Management of thoracic trauma victims. Philadelphia: Lippincott; 1980. p. 47–52.

[38] Ivatury RR. The injured heart. In: Moore EE, Feliciano DV, Mattox KL, editors. Trauma. 5th edition. New York: The McGraw-Hill Companies; 2004. p. 555–69.

THORACIC
SURGERY
CLINICS

ELSEVIER
SAUNDERS

Thorac Surg Clin 17 (2007) 11–23

Pulmonary Contusions and Critical Care Management in Thoracic Trauma

John P. Sutyak, EdM, MD[a,b,]*, Christopher D. Wohltmann, MD[a,b],
Jennine Larson, MD[b]

[a]*Southern Illinois Trauma Center, Southern Illinois University, P.O. Box 19663, Springfield, IL 62794, USA*
[b]*Department of Surgery, Southern Illinois University School of Medicine, P.O. Box 19663, Springfield, IL 62794, USA*

According to 2002 Centers for Disease Control and Prevention statistics, unintentional injury remains the leading cause of death for ages 1 through 44. Chest injuries are the primary cause in 9% of trauma mortalities and a likely contributor to the 28% of trauma mortality classified as "whole body system" by the Centers for Disease Control and Prevention [1]. Both blunt force and penetrating chest trauma can produce pulmonary dysfunction from multiple factors including direct lung injury, inhibition of chest wall movement, pressure on mediastinal structures, and systemic shock-activated inflammation. All of these factors compound the primary insult, causing secondary damage to initially uninjured lung. Isolated blunt pulmonary contusion is rare. More frequently, injury to the lung is part of multisystem trauma. In up to three quarters of cases, pulmonary contusions are associated with other local chest trauma, such as rib fractures, flail segments, and hemothoraces and pneumothoraces [2]. Pulmonary contusions are also frequently associated with nonthoracic trauma to the extremities, abdomen, and nervous system. Optimal treatment of patients with pulmonary and multisystem injuries requires the surgeon to recognize multiple, often conflicting, priorities in critical care management.

Treatment of pulmonary contusions and respiratory failure following trauma has advanced markedly in the past 60 years. The number of high-speed crashes increased with a proliferation of motor vehicle travel. As a result, chest injuries also increased in frequency. In the initial years following World War II, treatment of rib fractures and flail segments was based on external stabilization of the chest wall. Uncoordinated ventilation with resultant internal ventilatory shunting was believed to be the cause of respiratory failure after blunt chest trauma. In 1956, Avery and coworkers [3] introduced the concept of "internal pneumatic stabilization," which used positive pressure ventilation while awaiting adequate bony union. This application of mechanical ventilation along with the birth of critical care units resulted in improved outcomes; however, many complications continued to occur. In 1965, Reid and Baird [4] focused attention on the pulmonary tissue injury and not the rib cage instability. From the mid 1970s and into the 1980s, selective positive pressure ventilation for pulmonary support, not for chest wall stability, became standard therapy [5]. Current critical care for posttraumatic respiratory failure focuses on maintenance of adequate, not necessarily normal, pulmonary function; avoidance of iatrogenic injury; diligent treatment of infection; and patience for pulmonary tissue healing.

Pathophysiology of pulmonary contusion and ventilator-associated lung injury

Acute pulmonary dysfunction caused by trauma occurs on macroscopic and microscopic levels. Pathophysiologic changes occur within the entire thoracic cavity with such disorders as pneumothorax; massive lobar collapse (direct contusion or bronchial obstruction); and massive hemothorax.

---

* Corresponding author. Southern Illinois Trauma Center, Southern Illinois School of Medicine, P.O. Box 19663, Springfield, IL 62794.
  E-mail address: jsutyak@siumed.edu (J.P. Sutyak).

1547-4127/07/$ - see front matter © 2007 Elsevier Inc. All rights reserved.
doi:10.1016/j.thorsurg.2007.02.001

thoracic.theclinics.com

These disorders cause loss of large portions of lung, a mediastinal shift, and ventilation-perfusion mismatch. Correction through tube thoracostomy or bronchoscopy as appropriate is usually followed by clinical improvement.

A pulmonary contusion, either alone or in conjunction with other chest injury, also produces pulmonary dysfunction on the microscopic level. Numerous animal studies have increased understanding of the pathophysiology of pulmonary contusions. Following blunt force trauma to the chest, lacerations occur in the lung parenchyma [6]. These lacerations release blood and plasma that flood local alveoli. Local laceration combined with flooding of uninjured alveoli results in perfusion without ventilation, an increased intra-pulmonary shunt fraction, reduced compliance, increased pulmonary vascular resistance, reduced CO_2 elimination, and decreased oxygenation. The alveolar septa thicken as capillary leak occurs. These pathologic changes are not confined to the local zone of injury. Following unilateral experimental injury, effects occur in both lungs as demonstrated by histology, bronchoalveolar lavage (BAL) fluid examination, and assays of inflammatory markers [7–9]. The initial injury eventually reduces diffusion capacity in the uninjured lung. If the inflammatory response is of adequate magnitude, the result is a diffuse pulmonary dysfunction analogous to acute lung injury and acute respiratory distress syndrome (ARDS) with patches of normal functioning lung parenchyma interspersed with areas of consolidated fluid-filled nonfunctioning lung.

The clinical impact of the original process can be aggravated by the application of therapeutic positive pressure ventilation despite the best intentions and skill of physicians. The concept of barotrauma as a result of high pressure expansion of poorly compliant lung was previously confined to the development of extra-alveolar air. The broader hypothesis of ventilator-induced lung injury has been documented in multiple animal studies of injured and even normal lung [10–12]. Confirmation of direct ventilator-induced lung injury in humans is difficult because of many compounding clinical variables. Improved outcomes occur, however, with strategies aimed at preventing lung injury. It seems appropriate to at least adopt the concept of ventilator-associated lung injury even if direct human ventilator-induced injury has not been confirmed.

Barotrauma, volutrauma, atelectrauma, and biotrauma summarize important concepts in the pathophysiology of ventilator-associated lung injury [13–15]. These concepts should not be taken as isolated occurrences, but as synergistic and simultaneous effects of positive pressure on weakened lung tissue that is predisposed to additional injury. "Barotrauma" is the term most recognized by clinicians and refers to direct lung damage caused by excessive transpulmonary pressure. Air infiltrates the interstitial tissues and tracks along the bronchiovascular sheath. Pneumomediastinum, pneumopericardium, and subcutaneous emphysema are known results of barotrauma. If air ruptures into the pleural space, pneumothorax occurs. Many patients do not develop a classic pneumothorax as seen on chest radiographs. Fluid retained in the injured tissue prevents complete collapse. The effect of interstitial air can be critical, however, because it may impede the working, ventilated alveoli. On a microscopic level, disruption of the alveolar basement membrane occurs with bowing of alveolar borders, edema, and interstitial thickening.

Volutrauma refers to the injury produced by alveolar hyperdistention that may or may not be associated with increased pressure. In a whole rat model, isolated high volume with controlled pressure increases lung water. Isolated high pressure with controlled volume does not increase lung water [13,16]. The effects of excessive volume take place primarily in remaining normal lung tissue. Tidal volumes are diverted from the low compliance–high pressure injured alveoli to the higher compliance normal alveoli. Stretching and shear forces rupture both the endothelial and pneumocyte surfaces [13,17]. Interstitial and alveolar edema develops. More lung parenchyma loses diffusion capacity.

Repeated reopening of collapsed lung, even at low volumes, is also believed to play a role in ventilator-associated lung injury. This process has been labeled "atelectrauma" [13,15]. Repetitive recruitment and collapse produces significant injury on isolated nonperfused rat lungs [15,18]. When positive end-expiratory pressure (PEEP) is absent or below the threshold to maintain end-expiratory expansion, compliance decreases, and pathologic evidence of tissue damage is present. This does not occur when adequate PEEP is available to maintain postexpiratory volume. The damage caused by atelectrauma may be amplified by the miliary nature of lung injury. When areas of diseased lung are re-expanded, the surrounding areas of normal lung are subjected to extremely high regional pressures [15,19]. Once again, these forces lead to alveolar damage, leakage of interstitial fluid, and alveolar edema.

Barotrauma, volutrauma, and atelectrauma all refer to pneumatic mechanical stresses placed on the lung during positive pressure ventilation. Biotrauma describes the release of various inflammatory mediators during ventilator-associated lung injury. The mechanical factors may exert their continuing damage through this sustained inflammation. Animal studies of positive pressure ventilation have demonstrated elevated BAL and serum tumor necrosis factor-α (along with other cytokines), elevated arachidonic acid metabolites, and pulmonary neutrophilia [15,20–23]. These proinflammatory conditions were induced by volutrauma (high-volume ventilation or deliberate overinflation with PEEP); atelectrauma (no PEEP); and barotrauma (volume ventilation versus oscillatory ventilation). The effects of volutrauma and atelectrauma seem to be synergistic because cytokines increase dramatically with high-volume no-PEEP ventilation compared with either no PEEP or high volume alone [21]. Induced systemic proinflammatory mediators offer an explanation for the high incidence of end-stage multiple-system organ failure seen in severe respiratory failure. Current ventilator management aimed at reducing ventilator-associated lung injury has demonstrated lower mortality rates [24].

Support of pulmonary function

Currently, a direct method to speed repair of contused and secondarily injured pulmonary tissue does not exist. Therapy is based on support of oxygenation and ventilation with avoidance of further injury until spontaneous healing occurs and the patient is able to resume normal activities. Many therapeutic interventions exist to aide these vital functions. Understanding the options available, the capabilities and limits of each intervention, and their effects on pulmonary mechanics, gas exchange, and cardiac function is imperative for optimal patient management.

Noninvasive ventilation

Historically, noninvasive ventilation techniques consisted of either intermittent recruitment therapies, such as intermittent positive pressure breathing, or as ventilator-liberating facilitators, such as continuous positive airway pressure (CPAP). Over the past decade, however, noninvasive techniques have gained use in the primary treatment of patients with acute and chronic gas-exchange failure. Noninvasive positive pressure ventilation (NPPV), which delivers positive pressure in the form of CPAP or bi-level positive airway pressure (BiPAP), is safe and effective [25–27]. Other noninvasive support modes include nasal cannula and aerosol face mask. These modes support only oxygen exchange, whereas CPAP and BiPAP, as forms of NPPV, can be used to support both oxygenation and ventilation.

NPPV is delivered by a tight-fitting nasal or facemask and provides a set positive pressure for each breath without the need for an invasive airway. This allows for the conservation of normal speech, swallow, and cough mechanisms, but necessitates a cooperative patient. The primary role of NPPV is to facilitate secretion mobilization and treat atelectasis. It is generally well tolerated by patients and can be used intermittently or continuously. CPAP-BiPAP can be used with success to provide ventilator-free periods of support during acute respiratory distress in intubated patients. Cough and other bronchial hygiene techniques are essential components of positive airway pressure when the intent is secretion mobilization [28–30]. The application of positive airway pressure during NPPV improves oxygenation much like the addition of PEEP during conventional ventilation. By maintaining alveolar gas pressure and volume, NPPV increases pulmonary compliance and decreases work of breathing. In addition, NPPV has been found to decrease left ventricular afterload. It may also exert effects on preload, secondary to elevated intrathoracic pressures [31].

NPPV modes are widely applicable in critical care units, other acute inpatient units, or home care settings. The use of CPAP has been shown to decrease the incidence of endotracheal intubation and other respiratory complications in patients who develop hypoxemia postoperatively [32]. Proved applications for the use of CPAP or BiPAP include reducing air trapping in asthmatics or chronic obstructive pulmonary disease patients; mobilizing secretions; preventing or reducing atelectasis optimizing of bronchoactive medication delivery; relieving respiratory distress in cardiogenic pulmonary edema; and improving oxygenation in sepsis, acute lung injury, and ARDS [33–41]. Pure CPAP and BiPAP therapies require a spontaneously breathing patient and the ability adequately to monitor clinical response. All initiated breaths are patient driven. Minimally, patients should have subjective and physical evaluation of response to therapy, monitoring of oxygen saturation, blood gas analysis, vital signs, and chest radiographs (when clinically indicated). In the ICU setting, patients should be evaluated once hourly when using positive-pressure modes [42]. NPPV modes can be used in combination with bronchodilators and other respiratory adjuncts.

CPAP delivers continuous airway pressure during both inspiration and expiration. The patient breathes through a circuit against a threshold resistor that maintains a preset pressure from 5 to 20 cm H_2O. This pressure is maintained during inspiration as an external gas flow mechanism sufficient to sustain the desired positive airway pressure at the desired oxygen concentration [43–46]. Auto-CPAP systems have been developed. These devices adjust the pressure automatically to meet patient needs as breathing changes.

BiPAP differs from CPAP in that the pressure during expiration may be adjusted independent of the pressure during inspiration. The ability to titrate pressures independently during inspiration and expiration results in higher mean airway pressures than those produced using CPAP. BiPAP can function in a synchronized mode, a timed mode, or a combination mode. In the synchronized mode, BiPAP functions similarly to pressure support ventilation with CPAP. Pressure is coordinated and varies with the patient's respiratory cycle. In the timed mode, however, BiPAP provides ventilatory support on preset intervals, changing functional residual capacity during both inspiration and expiration. The patient performs inhalation and exhalation during both high- and low-pressure portions of the timed cycle. This effect is comparable with airway pressure release ventilation on intubated patients. The flexibility of BiPAP allows for both oxygenation and ventilatory support over a wide range of clinical situations [47]. Because BiPAP allows for independent adjustment of inspiratory and expiratory pressures, a trial of BiPAP may be useful in patients who cannot tolerate CPAP because of air hunger. Although initial patient acceptance may be higher with BiPAP, studies have failed to demonstrate increased hours of usage compared with CPAP [48].

There are several relative contraindications to the use of NPPV and situations in which special consideration should be given [49]. CPAP does not directly augment inspiration and may impede exhalation. This may lead to CO_2 retention in patients with ventilatory failure. Both CPAP and BiPAP increase air swallowing and can result in gastric distention, nausea, and emesis. The mask-delivery system may cause skin breakdown in areas of pressure or induce a sensation of suffocation or claustrophobia. Air leakage around the mask can occur, constraining effectiveness. Patients demonstrating a decreased level of consciousness or an inability to tolerate an increased work of breathing are at increased risk of developing hypoventilation and hypercarbia on NPPV. Elevations of intracranial pressure may occur and patients with an elevated intracranial pressure secondary to head trauma may not be candidates for higher pressure NPPV. Myocardial ischemia and decreased venous return induced by NPPV may preclude its use in patients with hemodynamic instability [50,51]. Judicious use in patients with an untreated pneumothorax, hemoptysis, maxillofacial trauma, or maxillofacial surgery is warranted before instituting mask NPPV. These potential pitfalls limit the use of CPAP and BiPAP to alert patients with mild to moderate respiratory failure. Overall, however, NPPV does offer a well-tolerated option for selected patients with acute respiratory failure [52].

Mechanical ventilation modes and lung protective strategies

Although the normal physiology of ventilation is based on the generation of negative intrathoracic pressure, pressure-cycled systems for positive pressure ventilation were the first to be used in mechanical ventilation. In pressure-cycled systems the pressure delivered is constant but the volume received is dependent on changes in lung mechanics. In contrast, volume-cycled systems function to deliver a constant, predetermined, alveolar volume regardless of lung mechanics. Currently, volume-controlled systems are the standard by which most positive-pressure mechanical ventilation is delivered [53,54].

Initially, large tidal volumes were used with positive pressure–volume-controlled ventilation in a belief that this prevented alveolar collapse. This belief has been supplanted by several studies demonstrating negative effects of large inflation volumes [13]. The notion of ventilator-associated lung injury has facilitated changes in the way that mechanical ventilation is delivered. A recent Acute Respiratory Distress Syndrome Network study was aimed at investigating lower tidal volumes and lung injury [24]. Tidal volumes of 6 and 12 mL/kg (based on calculated ideal body weight) were used to ventilate patients with ARDS. A significant absolute reduction in mortality was achieved using the lower tidal volumes and by maintaining end-inspiratory plateau pressure less than 30 cm H_2O. Improvements were noted even when the Pao_2 was slightly reduced and the $Paco_2$ elevated. Protective lung ventilation strategies often result in hypercapnia with respiratory acidosis. This is clinically acceptable to avoid the negative effects of high airway pressures. It is currently unclear if hypercapnia may actually be biologically protective against acute lung injury [55]. Low-volume and low-pressure ventilation is the current recommended strategy for patients with ARDS. Additional research efforts have also demonstrated a benefit from low-volume ventilation in other disease states [56].

Controlled mandatory ventilation

Assist-control or controlled mandatory ventilation is a mode of positive pressure, volume-controlled ventilation. This mode provides a minimum rate of set tidal volumes regardless of patient effort or breath initiation. Assist-control–controlled mandatory ventilation also allows the patient to initiate breaths above the minimum rate but delivers the same set tidal volume with each assisted breath. Typically, the inspiratory/expiratory ratio is at least 1:2. The trigger mechanism in assist-control–controlled mandatory ventilation may be flow or pressure based. Each trigger has its advantages and disadvantages that affect work of breathing. PEEP may be applied at end-expiration as needed to mitigate airway collapse and improve oxygen exchange. Adequate patient sedation during mechanical ventilation is important. Ventilatory drive is often increased in poorly sedated patients. This may lead to an increased work of breathing that can be reduced with improved patient comfort and sedation [57]. In patients with obstructive disease, high inflation volumes, rapid respiratory rates, or reduced expiratory volumes, air may be trapped at end-expiration, inducing a phenomenon known as "intrinsic" or "auto-PEEP" [58–60]. Unrecognized auto-PEEP may increase work of breathing, induce cardiac suppression, facilitate barotrauma, and spuriously increase central venous and cardiac filling pressures [61–63].

Intermittent mandatory ventilation

Originally developed for neonatal mechanical ventilation and to facilitate ventilator liberation, intermittent mandatory ventilation combines periods of assist-control ventilation with spontaneous breathing. Assisted breaths are synchronized with patient efforts, while maintaining a preset minute volume regardless of patient efforts. Periods of patient-driven ventilation reduce the development of intrinsic-PEEP and may maintain the strength of respiratory musculature. PEEP may be applied to improve oxygen exchange. As with assist-control modes, the trigger mechanism is either pressure or inspiratory flow regulated [64]. A potential disadvantage to intermittent mandatory ventilation is increased work of breathing, particularly in patients initiating numerous spontaneous breaths. Inspiratory pressure support can improve this by decreasing the mechanical resistance in the circuitry [65]. As with other forms of positive pressure ventilation, cardiac output and venous return can be reduced [66,67]. These are of added concern in patients with left ventricular dysfunction.

Pressure-controlled ventilation

In pressure-controlled ventilation (PCV), a pressure-limited breath is delivered at a minimum rate. Tidal volume is dependent on the peak pressure limit, inspiratory time, and compliance. The inspiratory flow pattern generated in PCV is always decelerating. Airflow slows as the pressure limit is approached. Volumes and airway pressures may be lower with PCV versus conventional volume-control ventilation [68]. The decelerating flow delivery may aid in preventing ventilator-associated lung injury through reduced peak pressure, increased static compliance, and improved gas distribution [69]. PCV has demonstrated use in ventilating patients with a significant air leak as in bronchopleural fistula [70,71]. Unlimited flow during inspiration that meets patient airflow demands is a major advantage of PCV. Prolonged inspiratory times and more rapid respiratory rates, however, increase the risk of auto-PEEP. Frequent operator adjustment is necessary in PCV. Because minute ventilation is not guaranteed and the inspiratory volumes are variable, patients must be monitored closely to avoid hypoventilation and hypoxia with changes in lung mechanics.

Pressure-regulated volume control ventilation

Pressure-regulated volume control ventilation is an A/C mode that combines volume ventilation with pressure limitation. The ventilator delivers guaranteed minute ventilation by adjusting inspiratory times and flow [72]. The level and time of pressure is continually varied to achieve the volume without exceeding the pressure limit. Volumes are augmented based on the most recent delivered. The theoretical advantage is avoidance of over distention while recruiting atelectatic alveoli. Compared with a straight volume control mode, such as A/C, pressure-regulated volume control ventilation provides a decelerating inspiratory flow pattern that produces lower peak inspiratory pressure without compromising volume [73].

Inverse ratio ventilation

Inverse ratio ventilation may be used in combination with PCV to enact prolonged inspiratory times. PCV–inverse ratio ventilation delivers a pressure-limited breath designed to facilitate recruitment of collapsed alveoli and prevent derecruitment. The normal inspiratory/expiratory ratio of 1:2 is increased, yielding reversed ratios of 1:1 up to 4:1. Prolonged inspiratory time theoretically delivers more uniform gas distribution with lower peak pressure. The real effects of inverse ratio ventilation, however, may be caused by increased PEEP occurring as auto-PEEP. A proved advantage of PCV–inverse ratio ventilation over modes using higher PEEP has not been demonstrated [74]. Typically, PCV–inverse ratio ventilation is reserved for patients with poor compliance and refractory hypoxemia, such as in ARDS and acute lung injury [75]. A serious limitation with inverse ratio ventilation is development of excessive auto-PEEP, which may produce cardiovascular compromise [76,77].

High-frequency oscillatory ventilation

High-frequency oscillation (HFO) ventilators generate low-amplitude proximal airway vibrations, analogous to acoustic waveforms, which result in sub-dead space tidal exchanges at varying airway pressures. HFO was initially used to treat respiratory failure in premature neonates. It has gained interest as a protective mode for ventilator-associated lung injury and as an option in refractory hypoxemia [78]. HFO has been used in the setting of acute lung injury and ARDS as both a primary and rescue mode [79]. It is presumed to reduce atelectrauma, the repetitive opening and closing of alveolar units. In HFO, airway pressure (analogous to BiPAP or airway pressure release ventilation), fraction of inspired oxygen, oscillatory frequency (analogous to rate), and amplitude (analogous to tidal volume) are titrated to achieve adequate oxygenation and ventilation.

Studies have failed to demonstrate significant improvements in outcome with HFO compared with other modes [75,80]. Significant improvements in oxygenation can be obtained, however, when HFO is used as a rescue in refractory hypoxemia [81]. Most patients on HFO require neuromuscular blockade to blunt spontaneous respiratory activity and improve tolerance. Cardiovascular compromise, breath "stacking," and pneumothorax are described side effects associated with HFO, but may be secondary to the disease state rather than the mode of ventilation [82].

Nitric oxide

Nitric oxide (NO) is a normal regulatory compound present in the vascular endothelium. Created by NO synthetase, NO increases cyclic GMP, relaxing vascular smooth muscle. Inhaled NO reduces pulmonary vascular resistance. NO acts locally and has an extremely short half-life of only a few seconds. The effects occur only on the vessels supplying ventilated functioning alveoli, not obstructed injured alveoli. Pulmonary blood flow is diverted into the dilated vessels resulting in a reduced shunt fraction, reduced ventilation-perfusion mismatch, and improved oxygenation. NO can be used alone or as an adjunct with prone positioning, HFO, or airway pressure release ventilation in patients with refractory hypoxemia. Dosage is started at 20 ppm and titrated down as the patient improves. Case reports of dramatic improvement and patient survival exist. Series have demonstrated only modest overall improvements in oxygenation, however, without significant reductions in mortality [83,84]. NO combines with oxygen to produce nitrogen dioxide (NO_2), an extremely toxic gas. The level of NO_2 and the NO/NO_2 ratio must be continuously monitored. When NO is metabolized to NO_2, NO also combines with water to create nitrite. These react with hemoglobin to produce methemoglobin. Methemoglobin cannot transport oxygen and levels must be monitored while a patient is receiving inhaled NO. Treatment for methemoglobinemia is 1% methylene blue, 1 to 2 mg/kg by slow IV infusion over 5 minutes.

Prone positioning

CT scan study of respiratory failure patients demonstrates that most collapse is in the posterior lung [85]. When a patient is supine in the ICU, most pulmonary blood flow is also posterior resulting in the highest flow to the poorest alveoli. Prone ventilation reverses this mismatch by returning pulmonary blood flow to the aerated alveoli in patients with severe hypoxemia. Limitations in using prone ventilation are primarily related to technical feasibility. Dislodgment of invasive devices, pressure damage, and positioning injuries constitute most of the risk of prone positioning. Specialty turning and padding equipment are available. Oxygenation can be increased; however, there has been no significant reduction in mortality [86]. The prone position increases intracranial pressure and is contraindicated in traumatic brain injury with elevated ICP [87,88].

Independent lung ventilation

Independent lung ventilation may be useful when a significant pathologic difference exists between lungs, and parallel ventilation fails. Independent lung ventilation indications include treatment of bronchopleural fistula; severe unilateral pulmonary disease (eg, aspiration); pulmonary embolus; or massive hemoptysis. A double-lumen endotracheal tube is placed with verification of position, typically by fiberoptic bronchoscopy. Two ventilators (conventional, jet, or high frequency) are then applied and adjusted as needed. Use of a double-lumen endotracheal tube increases the risk of airway trauma and reports of ischemia and bronchial rupture exist. Care must be taken in ensuring proper endotracheal tube size and position. Asynchronous independent lung ventilation is as effective as synchronous independent lung ventilation and generally well tolerated in adults. Advantages to an asynchronous approach include the option to apply different, unlinked, ventilators.

Ventilator-associated pneumonia

Ventilator-associated pneumonia (VAP) is the most frequent complication related to mechanical ventilation, occurring in 9% to 24% of patients with acute respiratory failure [89–91]. VAP accounts for almost 50% of acquired ICU infections [92]. Pneumonia is a leading cause of prolonged ICU stay (median of 6 days); hospital stay (9.2 days); and mortality (22%–42% increase) [90,91,93].

There are multiple risk factors for the development of VAP. The rate of pneumonia increases with the need for mechanical ventilation and continues to rise with increasing time on the ventilator at a rate of 1% to 3% per day [89]. Many patients with thoracic trauma have other associated injuries, such as intracerebral trauma, that predispose them to aspiration before intubation. Placement of an endotracheal tube facilitates passage of bacteria-laden oral flora into the bronchi. Airway reflexes are blunted and coughing is inhibited. The endotracheal tube cuff, properly inflated, does help to prevent aspiration but it is not a completely impervious barrier [93]. Oral secretions can pool and produce microaspiration [94]. Nasotracheal intubation is associated with a higher infection rate and mortality possibly caused by aspiration of infected sinus secretions [95]. All of these issues are compounded by the proinfection lung pathophysiology that develops following lung injury. Other risk factors for VAP include increasing injury severity score, decreasing Glasgow Coma Score, shock, and need for urgent intubation [96].

Diagnosis

Accurate diagnosis of VAP in the ICU patient can be challenging. The classic signs of pneumonia are new infiltrate on chest radiograph, fever, leukocytosis, and increased sputum production. Many chest trauma patients present with abnormal radiographs that make finding new infiltrates difficult. The multiply injured patient may have many possible sources for elevated temperature and white blood cell count. Amount and quality of sputum can be hard to assess. Gram stain and culture of endotracheal aspirates obtained by routine suctioning have been used to make the diagnosis of VAP. Multiple studies have shown that the analysis of these aspirates is often inaccurate and has many false-positives [97]. Administration of broad-spectrum antibiotics to treat these presumed pneumonias is harmful and has resulted in multidrug resistance [90].

BAL with quantitative culture has improved the accuracy of diagnosis and specificity of therapy in VAP. BAL obtains a more distal bronchial sample and prevents contamination by oral flora. The addition of quantitative culture allows for differentiation between colonization and infection. Based on the work of Croce and others [98,99], infection is indicated by the presence of at least 10^5 bacteria. The threshold may be lowered to at least 10^4 for *Pseudomonas* or *Acinetobacter* species. If the count is less than 10^5, antibiotics can be discontinued, because this count is indicative of colonization. Gram stain of the BAL effluent does not correlate well with the quantitative cultures, especially for gram-negative organisms, and should not be used to guide therapy [100]. BAL specimens are traditionally obtained by bronchoscopy. The proper equipment and clinical expertise may not be present at all institutions when the specimen is required. Other methods of obtaining bronchial samplings have been developed including "blind" bronchial brushing and protected telescoping catheters. These methods can be performed by respiratory therapists, and they have comparable results with bronchoscope-directed lavage [101–105].

Treatment

Early and aggressive treatment is required to improve the outcome in VAP [92,97,106]. Inadequate empiric antibiotic treatment results in increased morbidity and mortality [107]. Antibiotic therapy should be initiated after a BAL specimen is obtained. Continuation of antibiotic therapy should be based on the results of the BAL quantitative culture. The initial presumptive therapy should be broad, covering both gram-positive and -negative organisms. The antibiotic regimen should be tailored at 48 hours based on the culture results. In the first week, the predominant organisms are *Haemophilus* and gram-positive bacteria. After the first week, the nosocomial pathogens *Pseudomonas*, *Acinetobacter*, *Staphylococcus aureus*, and methicillin-resistant *S aureus* tend to appear [100]. Knowledge of the current local microflora and recent culture results can help determine the specific antibiotic selection.

Prevention

Invasive mechanical ventilation is known to increase the risk of pneumonia. Noninvasive ventilation and more rapid extubation should be beneficial. BiPAP and CPAP do decrease the rate of nosocomial pneumonia [108–110]. For intubated patients, adoption of daily weaning assessments and sedation protocols is associated with a decreased duration of intubation [111]. Sedation protocols should define clear targets for pain and anxiety relief. Daily spontaneous breathing trials in less critically ill patients should be performed. Care must be taken, however, not to extubate the patient prematurely. There is a clear increase in pneumonia in reintubated patients [112].

Secretions pool in the oropharyngeal and subglottic regions near the endotracheal tube cuff in an intubated patient. Bacterial overgrowth occurs in both locations. Secretion evacuation reduces overgrowth and, it is hoped, the incidence of microaspiration. Removal of secretions may also help to prevent formation of a biofilm around the endotracheal tube [94]. A subglottic drainage catheter on the endotracheal tube may prevent or delay the development of VAP [113].

Supine positioning places the mechanically ventilated patient at risk for aspiration and is an independent risk factor for VAP. Elevation of the head of the bed to 30% decreases rates of pneumonia and enteral nutrition aspiration [114–116]. This intervention is not as simple to achieve in trauma patients as it is in medical or other surgical patients. Spine stability must be considered when raising the head of the bed. External pelvic fixators and damage control abdominal dressings present additional challenges. If the patient cannot be flexed at the trunk because of spine instability, often the bed can be placed in a low Fowler's position (reverse Trendelenburg's) at 15 degrees to afford some advantage. Scheduled patient rotation is another method to avoid a continuously supine position. As with raising the head of the bed, spinal stability must be ensured. Many different kinetic beds have been developed and they decrease nursing work in turning. Use of these beds has decreased respiratory infection rates, but not ICU length of stay or ventilator days [93,117]. Another downside to kinetic beds is the increased cost.

The time-tested practice of hand washing before and after patient contact remains critically important for infection prevention. Good hand hygiene and the use of gloves helps to prevent patient-to-patient cross contamination and ventilator circuit contamination. Hand hygiene may be achieved with soap and water or hand sanitizers. Barrier gowns are appropriate when the patient is infected or colonized with certain multiresistant organisms, including methicillin-resistant *S aureus* [118,119]. There are no data indicating that the routine use of gowns for all ventilated patients results in a decreased pneumonia rate [120].

Stress ulcer prophylaxis has been used in mechanically ventilated patients because of a historical high rate of stress gastritis, ulcers, and upper gastrointestinal hemorrhage. The commonly used agents decrease gastric pH and may allow for gastric bacterial overgrowth. Initial studies suggested that sucralfate was a preferred agent, because it has no significant effect on pH. Recent studies have shown no increase in the pneumonia rate using histamine blockers. If a respiratory culture is positive in the presence of histamine antagonists, however, the organisms are more likely to be gram-negative bacteria [121]. There are no conclusive data regarding the relationship between proton pump inhibitors and the development of pneumonia.

Malnutrition decreases host immune functions and predisposes patients to infection. Nutritional support should be provided to a critically ill thoracic trauma patient once resuscitation is completed. Enteral nutrition is preferred to parenteral nutrition. There is no convincing evidence that jejunal feedings compared with gastric feedings reduce the rate of VAP [122]. Immune-enhancing enteral formulas have been proposed to improve the rates of VAP and overall ICU complications. Studies demonstrate a trend toward fewer infections compared with standard tube feeding formulas, but not a statistically significant improvement. These inconclusive data, coupled with the cost of immune-enhancing preparations, have prevented these formulas from becoming routine care [123].

Many or all of these prevention strategies should be incorporated into a ventilator care plan with a predefined ICU order set. This allows for standardization of physician, nursing, therapist, and dietician care.

References

[1] Miniño AM, Anderson RN, Fingerhut LA, et al. Deaths: injuries 2002. Natl Vital Stat Rep 2003; 54(10):1–128.

[2] Webb RR. Thoracic trauma. SCNA Newsl 1974; 54:1179–92.

[3] Avery EE, Morch ET, Benson DW. Critically crushed chests: a new method of treatment with continuous mechanical hyperventilation to produce alkalotic apnea and internal pneumatic stabilization. J Thorac Surg 1956;32:291–311.

[4] Reid JM, Baird WLM. Crushed chest injury: some physiological disturbances and their correction. Br Med J 1965;1:1105–9.

[5] Richardson JD, Adams L, Flint LM. Selective management of flail chest and pulmonary contusion. Ann Surg 1982;196:481–7.

[6] Oppenheimer L, Craven KD. Pathophysiology of pulmonary contusion in dogs. J Appl Physiol 1979;47:718–28.

[7] Hellinger A, Konerding MA. Does lung contusion affect both the traumatized and the noninjured lung parenchyma? A morphological and morphometric study in the pig. J Trauma 1995;39:712–9.

[8] Davis KA, Fabian TC. Prostanoids: early mediators in the secondary injury that develops after unilateral pulmonary contusion. J Trauma 1999; 46:824–31.

[9] Simon B, Ebert J, Bokhari F, et al. Practice management guideline for "pulmonary contusion – flail chest" June 2006. Eastern Association for the Surgery of Trauma. Available at: www.east.org. Accessed October 31, 2006.

[10] Dreyfuss D, Basset G, Soler P, et al. Intermittent positive-pressure hyperventilation with high inflation pressures produces pulmonary microvascular injury in rats. Am Rev Respir Dis 1985;132: 880–4.

[11] Kolobow T, Moreti MP, Fumigali R, et al. Severe impairment of lung function induced by high peak airway pressure during mechanical ventilation. Am Rev Respir Dis 1987;135:312–5.

[12] Tsuno K, Miura K, Takeya M, et al. Histopathologic pulmonary changes from mechanical ventilation at high peak airway pressures. Am Rev Respir Dis 1991;143:1115–20.

[13] Dreyfuss D, Saumon G. Ventilator-induced lung injury: lessons from experimental studies. Am J Respir Crit Care Med 1998;157:294–323.

[14] Dos Santos CC, Slutsky AS. The contribution of biophysical lung injury to the development of biotrauma. Annu Rev Physiol 2006;68:585–618.

[15] Slutsky AS. Lung injury caused by mechanical ventilation. Chest 1999;116:9S–15S.

[16] Dreyfuss D, Soler P, Basset G, et al. High inflation pressure pulmonary edema: respective effects of high airway pressure, high tidal volume, and positive end-expiratory pressure. Am Rev Respir Dis 1988;137:1159–64.

[17] Parker JC, Hernandez LA, Peevy KJ. Mechanisms of ventilator-induced lung injury. Crit Care Med 1993;21:131–43.

[18] Muscedere JG, Mullen J, Gan K, et al. Tidal ventilation at low airway pressures can augment lung injury. Am J Respir Crit Care Med 1994;149:1327–34.

[19] Mead J, Takishima T, Leith D. Stress distribution in lungs: a model of pulmonary elasticity. J Appl Physiol 1970;28:596–608.

[20] Imai Y, Kawano T, Miyasaka K, et al. Inflammatory chemical mediators during conventional ventilation and during high frequency oscillatory ventilation. Am J Resp Crit Care Med 1994;150: 1550–4.

[21] Tremblay L, Valenza F, Ribeiro SP, et al. Injurious ventilatory strategies increase cytokines and c-fos m-RNA expression in an isolated rat lung model. J Clin Invest 1997;99:944–52.

[22] Tremblay LN, Miatto D, Hamid Q, et al. Changes in cytokine expression secondary to injurious mechanical ventilation strategies in an ex vivo lung model. Intensive Care Med 1997;23(Suppl 1): S3.

[23] Ranieri VM, Suter PM, Tortorella D, et al. The effect of mechanical ventilation on pulmonary and systemic release of inflammatory mediators in patients with acute respiratory distress syndrome. JAMA 1999;282:54–61.

[24] The Acute Respiratory Distress Syndrome Network. Ventilation with lower tidal volumes as compared with traditional tidal volumes for acute lung injury and the acute respiratory distress syndrome. New Engl J Med 2000;342:1301–8.

[25] Keenan SP, Kernerman PD, Sibbald WJ, et al. Effect of noninvasive positive pressure ventilation on mortality in patients admitted with acute respiratory failure: a meta-analysis. Crit Care Med 1997; 25:1685–92.

[26] Nava S, Ambrosino N, Rubini F, et al. Noninvasive mechanical ventilation in the weaning of patients with respiratory failure due to chronic obstructive pulmonary disease: a randomized, controlled trial. Ann Intern Med 1998;128:721–8.

[27] Keenan SP, Sinuff T, Cook DJ, et al. Does noninvasive positive pressure ventilation improve outcome in acute hypoxemic respiratory failure? A systematic review. Crit Care Med 2004;32: 2516–23.

[28] Pavia D. The role of chest physiotherapy in mucus hypersecretion. Lung 1990;168(Suppl):614–21.

[29] Sutton PP, Lopez-Vidriero MT, Pavia D, et al. Assessment of percussion, vibratory-shaking and breathing exercises in chest physiotherapy. Eur J Respir Dis 1985;66(2):147–52.

[30] Navalesi P, Fanfulla F, Frigerio P, et al. Physiologic evaluation of non invasive mechanical ventilation delivered with three types of mask in patients with chronic hypercapnic respiratory failure. Crit Care Med 2000;28:1785–90.

[31] Lenique F, Habis M, Lofaso F, et al. Ventilatory and hemodynamic effects of continuous positive airway pressure in left heart failure. Am J Respir Crit Care Med 1997;155:500.

[32] Squadrone V, Coha M, Cerutti E, et al for the Piedmont Intensive Care Units Network (PICUN). Continuous positive airway pressure for treatment of postoperative hypoxemia: a randomized controlled trial. JAMA 2005;293:589–95.

[33] Petrof BJ, Calderini E, Gottfried SB. Effect of CPAP on respiratory effort and dyspnea during exercise in severe COPD. J Appl Physiol 1990;69(1): 179–88.

[34] Mansel JK, Stogner SW, Norman JR. Face-mask CPAP and sodium bicarbonate infusion in acute, severe asthma and metabolic acidosis. Chest 1989; 96:943–4.

[35] Martin JG, Shore S, Engel LA. Effect of continuous positive airway pressure on respiratory mechanics and pattern of breathing in induced asthma. Am Rev Respir Dis 1982;126:812–7.

[36] Hofmeyr JL, Webber BA, Hodson ME. Evaluation of positive expiratory pressure as an adjunct to chest physiotherapy in the treatment of cystic fibrosis. Thorax 1986;41(12):951–4.

[37] Kaminska TM, Pearson SB. A comparison of postural drainage and positive expiratory pressure in the domiciliary management of patients with chronic bronchial sepsis. Physiotherapy 1988; 74(5):251–4.

[38] Campbell T, Ferguson N, McKinlay RGC. The use of a simple self-administered method of positive expiratory pressure (PEP) in chest physiotherapy

after abdominal surgery. Physiotherapy 1986;72: 498–500.

[39] Ricksten SE, Bengtsson A, Soderberg C, et al. Effects of periodic positive airway pressure by mask on postoperative pulmonary function. Chest 1986;89:774–81.

[40] Confalonieri M, Potena A, Carbone G, et al. Acute respiratory failure in patients with severe community-acquired pneumonia: a prospective randomized evaluation of noninvasive ventilation. Am J Respir Crit Care Med 1999;160:1585–91.

[41] Peter JV, Moran JL, Phillips-Hughes J, et al. Effect of non-invasive positive pressure ventilation (NIPPV) on mortality in patients with acute cardiogenic pulmonary oedema: a meta-analysis. Lancet 2006;367(9517):1155–63.

[42] O'Dononue WJ Jr. Postoperative pulmonary complications: when are preventive and therapeutic measures necessary? Postgrad Med 1992;91: 167–70, 173–5.

[43] Carlsson C, Sonden B, Thylen U. Can postoperative continuous positive airway pressure (CPAP) prevent pulmonary complications after abdominal surgery? Intensive Care Med 1981;7:225–9.

[44] Garrard CS, Shah M. The effects of expiratory positive airway pressure on function residual capacity in normal subjects. Crit Care Med 1978;6:320–2.

[45] Lindner KH, Lotz P, Ahnefeld FW. Continuous positive airway pressure effect on functional residual capacity, vital capacity and its subdivisions. Chest 1987;92(1):66–70.

[46] Stock MC, Downs JB, Gauer PK, et al. Prevention of postoperative pulmonary complications with CPAP, incentive spirometry, and conservative therapy. Chest 1985;87:151–7.

[47] International Consensus Conferences in Intensive Care Medicine: noninvasive positive pressure ventilation in acute respiratory failure. Am J Respir Crit Care Med 2001;163(1):283–91.

[48] Reeves-Hoche MK, Hudgel DW, Meck R, et al. Continuous versus bilevel positive airway pressure for obstructive sleep apnea. Am J Respir Crit Care Med 1995;151(2):443–9.

[49] Mahlmeister MJ, Fink JB, Hoffman GL, et al. Positive-expiratory-pressure mask therapy: theoretical and practical considerations and a review of the literature. Respir Care 1991;36(11):1218–30.

[50] Fessler HR, Brower R, Wise R, et al. Mechanism of reduced LV afterload by systolic and diastolic positive pleural pressure. J Appl Physiol 1988;65: 1244–50.

[51] Katz JA, Marks JD. Inspiratory work with and without continuous positive airway pressure in patients with acute respiratory failure. Anesthesiology 1985;63:598–607.

[52] Hill NS. Complications of noninvasive positive pressure ventilation. Respir Care 1997;42:432–42.

[53] Fan E, Needham DM, Stewart TE. Ventilatory management of acute lung injury and acute

respiratory distress syndrome. JAMA 2005;294: 2889–96.

[54] Tobin MJ. Advances in mechanical ventilation. N Engl J Med 2001;344:1986–96.

[55] O' Croninin D, Ni Chonghaile M, Higgins B, et al. Bench-to-bedside review: permissive hypercapnia. Crit Care 2005;9(1):51–9 [Epub 2004 Aug 5].

[56] Gajic O, Dara D, Mendez JL, et al. Ventilator-associated lung injury in patients without acute lung injury at the onset of mechanical ventilation. Crit Care Med 2004;32:1817–24.

[57] Fernandez R, Blanch L, Antigas A. Respiratory center activity during mechanical ventilation. J Crit Care 1991;6:102–11.

[58] Pepe P, Marini JJ. Occult positive end-expiratory pressure in mechanically ventilated patients with airflow obstruction. Am Rev Respir Dis 1982;126: 166–70.

[59] Leatherman JW, Ravenscraft SA. Low measured auto-positive end-expiratory pressure during mechanical ventilation of patients with severe asthma: hidden auto-positive end-expiratory pressure. Crit Care Med 1996;24(3):541–6.

[60] Moore FA, Haenel JB, Moore EE, et al. Auto-PEEP in the multisystem injured patient: an elusive complication. J Trauma 1990;30(11):1316–22 [discussion: 1322–3].

[61] Patroniti N, Pesenti A. Low tidal volume, high respiratory rate and auto-PEEP: the importance of the basics. Crit Care 2003;7(2):105–6 [Epub 2003 Jan 31].

[62] Teboul JL, Pinsky MR, Mercat A, et al. Estimating cardiac filling pressures in mechanically ventilated patients with hyperinflation. Crit Care Med 2000; 28:3631–6.

[63] Sydow M, Golisch W, Burchardi H, et al. Effect of low-level PEEP on inspiratory work of breathing in intubated patients, both with healthy lungs and with COPD. Intensive Care Med 1995;21(11): 887–95.

[64] Leung P, Jubran A, Tobin MJ. Comparison of assisted ventilator modes on triggering, patient effort, and dyspnea. Am J Respir Crit Care Med 1997;155(6):1940–8.

[65] Shelledy DC, Rau JL, Thomas-Goodfellow L. A comparison of the effects of assist-control, SIMV, and SIMV with pressure support on ventilation, oxygen consumption, and ventilatory equivalent. Heart Lung 1995;24(1):67–75.

[66] Sternberg R, Sahebjami H. Hemodynamic and oxygen transport characteristics of common ventilatory modes. Chest 1994;105(6):1798–803.

[67] Pinsky MR. Cardiovascular issues in respiratory care. Chest 2005;128(Suppl):592S–7S.

[68] Cinnella G, Conti G, Lofaso F, et al. Effects of assisted ventilation on the work of breathing: volume-controlled versus pressure-controlled ventilation. Am J Respir Crit Care Med 1996;153(3): 1025–33.

[69] Rappaport SH, Shpiner R, Abraham E, et al. Randomized, prospective trial of pressure-limited versus volume-controlled ventilation in severe respiratory failure. Crit Care Med 1994;22(1): 22–32.

[70] Paulson TE, Spear RM, Silva PD, et al. High-frequency pressure-control ventilation with high positive end-expiratory pressure in children with acute respiratory distress syndrome. J Pediatr 1996;129(4):566–73.

[71] Munoz J, Guerrero JE, Escalante JL, et al. Pressure-controlled ventilation versus controlled mechanical ventilation with decelerating inspiratory flow. Crit Care Med 1993;21(8):1143–8.

[72] Macintyre NR, Gropper C, Wesfall T. Combining pressure-limiting and volume-cycling features in a patient-interactive mechanical breath. Crit Care Med 1994;22(2):353–7.

[73] Guldager H, Soeren LN, Peder C, et al. A comparison of volume control and pressure-regulated volume control ventilation in acute respiratory failure. Crit Care 1997;1:75–7.

[74] Neumann P, Berglund JE, Andersson LG, et al. Effects of inverse ratio ventilation and positive end-expiratory pressure in oleic acid-induced lung injury. Am J Respir Crit Care Med 2000; 161:1537–45.

[75] Tharratt RS, Allen RP, Albertson TE. Pressure controlled inverse ratio ventilation in severe adult respiratory failure. Chest 1988;94(4):755–62.

[76] Schreiter D, Reske A, Josten C, et al. Alveolar recruitment in combination with sufficient positive end-expiratory pressure increases oxygenation and lung aeration in patients with severe chest trauma. Crit Care Med 2004;32(4):968–75.

[77] Wang SH, Wei TS. The outcome of early pressure-controlled inverse ratio ventilation on patients with severe acute respiratory distress syndrome in surgical intensive care unit. Am J Surg 2002;183(2): 151–5.

[78] Bhuta T, Henderson-Smart DJ. Elective high-frequency oscillatory ventilation versus conventional ventilation in preterm infants with pulmonary dysfunction: systematic review and meta-analyses. Pediatrics 1997;100:1–7.

[79] Mehta S, Lapinsky SE, Hallett DC, et al. Prospective trial of high-frequency oscillation in adults with acute respiratory distress syndrome. Crit Care Med 2001;29:1360–9.

[80] Wunsch H, Mapstone J. High-frequency ventilation versus conventional ventilation for treatment of acute lung injury and acute respiratory distress syndrome. Cochrane Database Syst Rev 2004;1: CD004085.

[81] Derdak S, Mehta S, Stewart TE, et al. High-frequency oscillatory ventilation for acute respiratory distress syndrome in adults: a randomized, controlled trial. Am J Respir Crit Care Med 2002; 166:801–8.

[82] Mehta S, Granton J, MacDonald RJ, et al. High-frequency oscillatory ventilation in adults: the Toronto experience. Chest 2004;126:518–27.

[83] Taylor RW, Zimmerman JL, Dellinger RP, et al. Low-dose inhaled nitric oxide in patients with acute lung injury: a randomized controlled trial. JAMA 2004;291:1603–9.

[84] Levy B, Bollaert PE, Larcan A. Inhaled nitric oxide is often efficient in severe ARDS. Intensive Care Med 1995;21(10):864.

[85] Gattinoni LD, Mascheroni A, Torresin R, et al. Morphological response to positive end-expiratory pressure in acute respiratory failure: computerized tomography study. Intensive Care Med 1986;12:137–42.

[86] Pelosi P, Brazzi L, Gattinoni L, et al. Prone position in acute respiratory distress syndrome. Eur Respir J 2002;20:1017–28.

[87] Guerin C, Gaillard S, Lemasson S, et al. Effects of systematic prone positioning in hypoxemic acute respiratory failure: a randomized controlled trial. JAMA 2004;292:2379–87.

[88] Staudinger T, Kofler J, Mullner M, et al. Comparison of prone positioning and continuous rotation of patients with adult respiratory distress syndrome: results of a pilot study. Crit Care Med 2001;29:51–6.

[89] Rakshit P, Nagar VS, Deshpande AK. Incidence, clinical outcome, and risk stratification of ventilator-associated pneumonia: a prospective cohort study. Indian Journal of Critical Care Medicine 2005;9:211–6.

[90] Fagon JY, Chastre J, Domart Y, et al. Nosocomial pneumonia in patients receiving continuous mechanical ventilation: prospective analysis of 52 episodes with use of a protected specimen brush and quantitative culture techniques. Am Rev Respir Dis 1989;139:877–84.

[91] Torres A, Aznar R, Gatell JM, et al. Incidence, risk, and prognosis factors of nosocomial pneumonia in ventilated patients. Am Rev Respir Dis 1990;142:523–8.

[92] Chastre J, Luyt C, Combes A, et al. Use of quantitative cultures and reduced duration of antibiotic regimens for patients with ventilator-associated pneumonia to decrease resistance in the intensive care unit. Clin Infect Dis 2006;43(Suppl 2):75–81.

[93] Ferrer R, Artigas A. Clinical review: non-antibiotic strategies for preventing ventilator-associated pneumonia. Crit Care 2002;6(1):45–51.

[94] Safdar N, Crnich CJ, Maki DG. The pathogenesis of ventilator-associated pneumonia: its relevance to developing effective strategies for prevention. Respir Care 2005;50(6):725–39.

[95] Rouby JJ, Laurent P, Gosnach M, et al. Risk factors and clinical relevance of nosocomial maxillary sinusitis in the critically ill. Am J Respir Crit Care Med 1994;150:776–83.

[96] Croce MA, Fabian TC, Waddle-Smith L, et al. Identification of early predictors for post-traumatic pneumonia. Am Surg 2001;67:105–10.

[97] Meduri GU, Wunderink RG, Leeper KV, et al. Management of bacterial pneumonia in ventilated patients: protected bronchoalveolar lavage as a diagnostic tool. Chest 1992;101(2):500–8.

[98] Croce MA, Tolley EA, Fabian TC. A formula for prediction of posttraumatic pneumonia based on early anatomic and physiologic parameters. J Trauma 2003;54:724–30.

[99] Croce MA, Fabian TC, Mueller EW, et al. The appropriate diagnostic threshold for ventilator-associated pneumonia using quantitative cultures. J Trauma 2004;56:931–6.

[100] Croce MA, Fabian TC, Waddle-Smith L, et al. Utility of Gram's stain and efficacy of quantitative cultures for posttraumatic pneumonia. Ann Surg 1998;227(5):743–55.

[101] Bello S, Tajada A, Chacon E, et al. Blind protected specimen brushing versus bronchoscopic techniques in the aetiological diagnosis of ventilator-associated pneumonia. Eur Respir J 1996;9(7):1339–41.

[102] Marik PE, Careau P. A comparison of mini-bronchoalveolar lavage and blind-protected specimen brush sampling in ventilated patients with suspected pneumonia. J Crit Care 1998;13(2):67–72.

[103] Wood AY, Davit AJ, Ciraulo DL, et al. A prospective assessment of diagnostic efficacy of blind protective bronchial brushings compared to bronchoscope-assisted lavage, bronchoscope-directed brushings, and blind endotracheal aspirates in ventilator-associated pneumonia. J Trauma 2003;55(5):825–34.

[104] Mentec H, May-Michelangeli L, Rabbat A, et al. Blind and bronchoscopic sampling methods in suspected ventilator-associated pneumonia: a multicentre prospective study. Intensive Care Med 2004;30(7):1319–26.

[105] Rajasekhar T, Anuradha K, Suhasini T, et al. The role of quantitative cultures of non-bronchoscopic samples in ventilator-associated pneumonia. Indian J Med Microbiol 2006;24(2):107–13.

[106] Mehta RM, Niederman MS. Nosocomial pneumonia. Curr Opin Infect Dis 2002;15(4):387–94.

[107] Mueller EW, Hanes SD, Croce MA, et al. Effect from multiple episodes of inadequate empiric antibiotic therapy for ventilator-associated pneumonia on morbidity and mortality among critically ill trauma patients. J Trauma 2005;58:94–101.

[108] Tablan OC, Anderson LJ, Besser R, et al. CDC Healthcare Infection Control Practices Advisory Committee. Guidelines for preventing healthcare-associated pneumonia 2003: recommendations of CDC and the Healthcare Infection Control

Practices Advisory Committee. MMWR Recomm Rep 2004;53(RR-3):1–36.

[109] Nourdine K, Comes P, Carton MJ, et al. Does non-invasive ventilation reduce the ICU nosocomial infection risk? A prospective clinical survey. Intensive Care Med 1999;25:567–73.

[110] Girou E, Schortgen F, Delclaux C, et al. Association of noninvasive ventilation with nosocomial infections and survival in critically ill patients. JAMA 2000;284:2361–76.

[111] Kress JP, Pohlman AS, O'Connor MF, et al. Daily interruption of sedative infusions in critically ill patients undergoing mechanical ventilation. N Engl J Med 2000;342:1471–7.

[112] de Lassence A, Alberti C, Azoulay E, et al. OUT-COMEREA Study Group. Impact of unplanned extubation and reintubation after weaning on nosocomial pneumonia risk in the intensive care unit: a prospective multicenter study. Anesthesiology 2002;97(1):148–56.

[113] Iregui M, Kollef M. Prevention of ventilator-associated pneumonia selecting interventions that make a difference. Chest 2002;121:679–81.

[114] Torres A, Serra battles J, Ros E, et al. Pulmonary aspiration of gastric contents in patients receiving mechanical ventilation: the effect of body position. Ann Intern Med 1992;116:540–3.

[115] Orozco-Levi M, Torres A, Ferrer M, et al. Semirecumbent position protects from pulmonary aspiration but not completely from gastroesophageal reflux in mechanically ventilated patients. Am J Respir Crit Care Med 1995;152:1387–90.

[116] Drakulovic M, Torres A, Bauer TT, et al. Supine position is a risk factor of nosocomial pneumonia in mechanically ventilated patients: a randomized clinical trial. Lancet 1999;354:1851–8.

[117] Delaney A, Gray H, Laupland KB, et al. Kinetic bed therapy to prevent nosocomial pneumonia in mechanically ventilated patients: a systemic review and meta-analysis. Crit Care 2006;10(3):R70.

[118] Bearman GM, Munro C, Sessler CN, et al. Infection control and the prevention of nosocomial infections in the intensive care unit. Semin Respir Crit Care Med 2006;27(3):310–24.

[119] Girou E. Prevention of nosocomial infections in acute respiratory failure patients. Eur Respir J Suppl 2003;42:72s–6s.

[120] Koss WG, Khalili TM, Lemus JF, et al. Nosocomial pneumonia is not prevented by protective contact isolation in the surgical intensive care unit. Am Surg 2001;67(12):1140–4.

[121] Thomason MH, Payseur ES, Hakenewerth AM, et al. Nosocomial pneumonia in ventilated trauma patients during stress ulcer prophylaxis with sucralfate, antacid, and ranitidine. J Trauma 1996;41(3):503–8.

[122] Marik PE, Zaloga GP. Gastric versus post-pyloric feeding: a systematic review. Crit Care 2003;7(3):R46–51.

[123] Montejo JC, Zarazaga A, Lopez-Martinez J, et al. Spanish Society of Intensive Care Medicine and Coronary Units. Immunonutrition in the intensive care unit. A systematic review and consensus statement. Clin Nutr 2003;22(3):221–33.

ELSEVIER
SAUNDERS

Thorac Surg Clin 17 (2007) 25–33

THORACIC
SURGERY
CLINICS

The Management of Flail Chest

Brian L. Pettiford, MD, James D. Luketich, MD,
Rodney J. Landreneau, MD*

*Heart, Lung and Esophageal Surgery Institute, University of Pittsburgh Medical Center,
Shadyside Medical Center, Suit 715, 5200 Centre Avenue, Pittsburgh, PA 15232, USA*

Thoracic trauma is quite common in the United States, with a broad injury profile that ranges from abrasions and contusions to aortic transection with exsanguinating hemorrhage. The cause of thoracic trauma is legion and includes motor vehicle crashes, assaults, falls, occupational-related crush accidents, and sports injuries. Motor vehicle crash accounts for over 43,000 accidental injuries in the United States each year [1]. It is the most common cause of thoracic trauma, accounting for nearly 80% of reported chest wall injuries in some series [2,3]. Thoracic trauma has serious implications, accounting for nearly 20% of all trauma deaths in the United States [4].

Most thoracic injury sustained in motor vehicle crash is blunt in nature [5]. The three main types of blunt injury forces are (1) compression, (2) shearing, and (3) blast. Steering wheel contact with the thoracic cage contributes to compressive chest wall or thoracic organ injury. Acute deceleration from a head-on or lateral impact motor vehicle crash may cause a shearing injury. This force may also occur after a fall and may lead to aortic transection. The concussive force from a blast is most commonly associated with high-energy explosives usually seen in a military setting. The distance between the victim and the blast epicenter may affect the extent of injury [6]. Large stationary objects between the victim and the blast source may absorb a considerable amount of energy and subsequently decrease the extent of injury.

Pathophysiology

A common result of compressive injury to the thoracic cage is rib fracture. The fracture location is influenced by the angle of impact. Rib fractures tend to occur anteriorly at 60-degree rotation from the sternum [7]. Frontal and lateral impact, however, may result in multiple anterior and posterior rib fracture points. Severe anterior compressive forces may cause sternochondral disruption and a subsequent sternal flail. Flail chest occurs in 10% of thoracic trauma cases and has a reported mortality rate between 10% and 15% [2,8–10].

Flail chest is defined as the fracture of four or more consecutive ribs in at least two places. This is accompanied by paradoxical motion of the affected chest wall segment during respiration such that the flail segment collapses during inspiration and expands during expiration (Fig. 1). During inspiration, the flail segment decreases the negative intrathoracic forces required for adequate ipsilateral lung expansion. The lateral motion of the flail segment lessens the positive intrathoracic pressure needed during expiration. Flail chest can be subdivided into anterior and posterior flail chest depending on the presence of fractures along the anterior or posterior rib angles, respectively (Fig. 2). Borrelly and Aazami [11] reported that contraction of the serratus anterior muscle digitations pulls the flail segment posteriorly and superiorly. Canine flail chest experiments have also shown that the degree of inward inspiratory displacement is related to force differences between intrapleural pressure and parasternal muscle activity [12].

Initial evaluation

The diagnosis of flail chest is clinical and requires evaluation of the injury mechanism,

---

* Corresponding author.
E-mail address: landreneaurj@upmc.edu
(R.J. Landreneau).

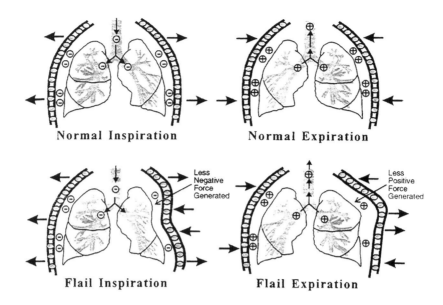

Fig. 1. Schematic of flail chest physiology. (*From* Mayberry J, Trunkey D. The fractured rib in chest wall trauma. Chest Surg Clin N Am 1997;7:253; with permission.)

physical examination, and radiographic studies including plain film chest radiograph. With regard to injury mechanism, motor vehicle crash is a major contributor to the development of flail chest. Emergency medical personnel reports of steering wheel deformity, high speed frontal or lateral crash, and the presence or absence of front and side airbags is useful during patient triage.

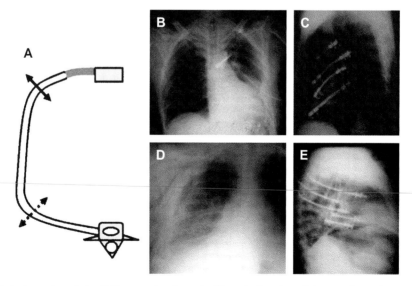

Fig. 2. (*A*) Anterior and posterior flail segments schematic. Note the location of the anterior and posterior fractures along the anterior and posterior rib angles, respectively. (*B, C*) Preoperative and postoperative chest radiograph of antero-lateral flail segment. (*D, E*) Preoperative and postoperative chest radiograph of posterolateral flail segment. (*From* Borrelly J, Aazami M. New insights into the pathophysiology of flail segment: the implication of anterior serratus muscle in parietal failure. Eur J Cardiothor Surg 2005;28:743; with permission. Copyright © 2005, European Organization for Cardio-Thoracic Surgery.)

Shoulder harness seatbelt use may also provide information about the possibility of sternal or rib fracture versus chest wall contusion.

Patients with flail chest should undergo a standard initial trauma resuscitation including airway, breathing, and circulation assessment. Physical examination generally reveals a paradoxical motion of the flail chest wall segment with normal respiration. The flail segment becomes depressed with inspiration and moves laterally with expiration. The awake patient usually complains of severe chest wall pain and may manifest signs of respiratory insufficiency including tachypnea and splinting. Decreased breath sounds may indicate a pneumothorax, pulmonary contusion, or hemothorax. Radiographic evaluation begins with a portable anteroposterior chest radiograph. This may not reveal an underlying rib fracture along the lateral and more posterior aspects of the rib. Given the severity of the accident and concomitant intra-abdominal injuries, most patients undergo a chest and abdominal CT scan. This study better identifies rib fractures and further defines additional intrathoracic injury, such as aortic dissection-transection, hemothorax, and anterior pneumothorax.

Medical management

The initial management of flail chest focuses primarily on maintaining adequate ventilation. Intermittent positive pressure ventilation was first successfully used to manage flail chest in the mid 1950s [13]. Cullen and colleagues [14] further supported the use of intermittent mechanical ventilation in the treatment of flail chest. During the late 1960s and early 1970s, flail chest was managed with early tracheostomy and mechanical ventilation. It was believed that the hypoxia, decreased compliance, increased work of breathing, and decline in pulmonary function testing were solely caused by the flail segment. At that time, only the paradoxical motion of the flail segment characterized flail chest, with no consideration for underlying pulmonary contusion [15–17]. Trinkle and colleagues [18], however, recommended primary treatment of the underlying lung injury with a combination of fluid restriction, corticosteroids, aggressive pulmonary toilet, and pain control. They described a decrease in mortality rate from 21% to 0%, a 5-fold decrease in morbidity, and a nearly 3.5-fold decrease in hospital stay in these patients when compared with those undergoing tracheostomy and mechanical ventilation.

At present, most patients with isolated flail chest are admitted to a trauma ICU and receive aggressive pulmonary toilet and pain control. In patients with an isolated flail chest injury, adequate analgesia greatly facilitates pulmonary toilet and early patient mobilization. Systemic opioids, such as intravenous fentanyl or morphine sulfate, may provide adequate pain relief. Patient-controlled anesthesia is also effective. Patient-controlled anesthesia with a continuous infusion has been shown to improve pain scores; however, respiratory depression may result. Bupivacaine intercostal nerve block is useful for pain management of isolated rib fracture. Multiple rib fractures require several injections, however, and may result in additional chest wall pain, pneumothorax, and even local anesthetic toxicity [19].

Epidural analgesia has proved extremely effective in managing the acute pain from chest wall injury. Splinting and paradoxical chest wall motions are improved to near normal levels. Epidural use improves pulmonary toilet by enabling the patient to breathe deeply, cough effectively, and actively participate in chest physiotherapy [20–22]. Adverse effects, such as hypotension in the underresuscitated patient, respiratory depression, and epidural infection, can limit its effectiveness [21]. In addition, epidurals can hinder diagnosis of intra-abdominal injuries in critically ill trauma patients [23]. Despite these potential complications, epidural analgesia remains central in the management of flail chest.

Thoracic paravertebral block is a technique whereby local anesthetic is injected along the thoracic vertebrae. This modality provides ipsilateral analgesia over a dermatomal distribution and, unlike epidural anesthesia, minimizes hypotension secondary to a unilateral sympathetic blockade [24–26]. Nonsteroidal anti-inflammatory drugs, such as ketorolac and indomethacin, are effective in the management of mild to moderate chest wall pain. They are particularly useful when used as an adjunct to patient-controlled anesthesia or epidural analgesia. Nonsteroidal anti-inflammatory drug use is limited in many trauma patients who may have acute renal failure or stress gastric ulcers.

Outcome and prognosis

The high mortality rate is primarily caused by associated injuries, such as pulmonary contusion and intra-abdominal or intracranial injury. In one series, 100% mortality was observed in patients with flail chest and concomitant head injuries [27].

The Injury Severity Score has been a useful marker for determining the effects of associated injuries on outcome in patients with flail chest. An increased Injury Severity Score has been related to an increased morbidity and mortality in patients with flail chest [2,27].

Early mechanical ventilatory assistance is provided to patients with severe concomitant injuries. An Injury Severity Score greater than 23, head or truncal organ injury, shock on admission, and blood transfusions within the first 24 hours have all been associated with the need for mechanical ventilation. The mortality rate of patients with severe associated injuries may be decreased from 50% to 6% if mechanical ventilation is instituted within 24 hours of injury. The mortality rate can exceed 90%, however, for patients with flail chest and hypotension who develop hypoxia for a period of more than 24 hours [27].

Internal pneumatic stabilization may allow for fibrous chest wall stability. In addition, pulmonary toilet can be provided by flexible bronchoscopy. Even so, the incidence of pneumonia progressively increases with the duration of intubation and mechanical assistance [28]. Other pneumatic stabilization measures, such as continuous positive airway pressure (CPAP), may decrease atelectasis in awake, spontaneously breathing patients and improve outcome in the critically ill and in trauma patients [29–31]. In a prospective randomized study comparing CPAP with mechanical ventilation with intermittent positive pressure ventilation, Gunduz and colleagues [32] demonstrated a lower mortality and lower nosocomial infection rate. There was no difference in oxygenation and ICU length of stay. The authors supported the use of CPAP as initial treatment of flail chest.

Some patients with flail chest progress to develop respiratory failure manifested by an increased work of breathing, progressive hypoxemia, and hypercarbia. Other patients have serious concomitant injuries, such as brain trauma, that dictate intubation and mechanical ventilation. Those patients who are mechanically ventilated may be maintained on synchronized intermittent mandatory ventilation setting with pressure support or positive end-expiratory pressure if their hemodynamic status permits. Patients with flail chest and pulmonary contusion may develop a clinical profile similar to acute respiratory distress syndrome, with progressive hypoxemia, elevated airway pressures, and a progressive infiltrate in the affected lung. Pulmonary contusion increases risk for the development of pneumonia and is associated with prolonged mechanical ventilation and higher mortality rate in flail chest victims [33,34]. Functional residual capacity is also decreased in flail chest patients who survive pulmonary contusions [35]. A subset of these patients become progressively more difficult to oxygenate and may require pressure control ventilation. Combined differential lung ventilation with inhaled nitric oxide may also be used in the management of flail chest complicated by severe pulmonary contusion [36]. Extracorporeal membranous oxygenation may be used in isolated cases of pulmonary contusion that is refractory to the previously mentioned measures [37–39]. Such factors as intracranial hemorrhage, sepsis, and poor overall prognosis limit the use of this therapeutic modality. Treatment of patients with flail chest and severe pulmonary contusion is difficult. Prolonged mechanical ventilation with early tracheostomy is the rule when managing this patient group.

Surgical management

The surgical management of flail chest has traditionally been reserved for the following indications: (1) patients with flail chest who require thoracotomy for other intrathoracic injury, (2) those who are unable to be successfully weaned from mechanical ventilatory assistance, (3) severe chest wall instability, (4) persistent pain secondary to fracture malunion, and (5) persistent or progressive loss of pulmonary function [40,41]. Landreneau and colleagues [42] demonstrated that Luque rod strut fixation of extensive flail chest resulted in restoration of normal volume of the affected hemithorax. This external fixation approach allowed for successful ventilator weaning after several weeks of continued ventilator support (Fig. 3). Furthermore, the strut fixation apparatus was easily removed at the bedside using minimal sedation. Tanaka and colleagues [43], in a randomized prospective study of surgical versus internal pneumatic stabilization of flail chest, demonstrated less ventilatory support, low pneumonia incidence, and a shorter ICU stay in patients undergoing surgical stabilization. Furthermore, surgical stabilization was associated with a lower medical cost and a faster return to employment.

Internal fixation techniques including plate stabilization, wire cerclage, intramedullary fixation, and vertical bridging have all been used in the management of flail chest. Haasler [44]

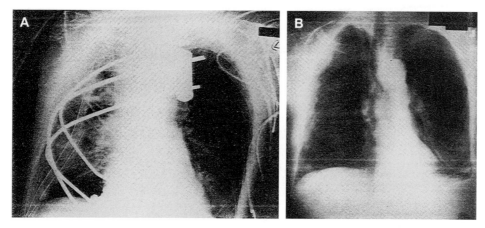

Fig. 3. (*A*) Chest radiograph of Luque rod fixation of posterolateral flail chest stabilized with orthopedic external fixation devices. (*B*) Plain film approximately 3 months after device removal. (*From* Landreneau R, Hinson J, Hazelrigg S, et al. Strut fixation of an extensive flail chest. Ann Thorac Surg 1991;51:474; with permission. Copyright © 1991, The Society of Thoracic Surgeons.)

performed an open fixation using Adkins struts to stabilize the anterior and posterior fractures in a patient with flail chest and refractory dyspnea with minimal exertion (Fig. 4). The patient had resolution of her symptoms with normalization of her pulmonary function testing profile at 1 year postoperatively. Judet struts and acetabular reconstruction plates may be used to provide internal fixation (Fig. 5). Oyarzun and colleagues [45] described a technique of operative stabilization using 3.5-mm acetabular reconstruction plates. The plates are contoured appropriately and secured along the long axis of the rib using cortical screws (Figs. 6 and 7). Special care is taken to avoid neurovascular bundle injury. The main advantages of this technique are the speed of implantation and that plate extraction is not generally required.

A possible disadvantage of the metal prosthesis is that it absorbs most of the stress directed toward the affected rib, potentially resulting in delayed fracture healing. Furthermore, the rigidity of metal prostheses exceeds that of the affected ribs and may result in screw loosening, plate dislocation, or chronic chest wall pain, requiring subsequent removal [46]. Absorbable polylactide

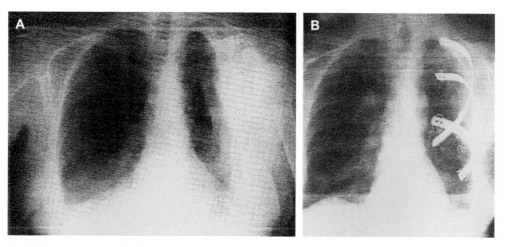

Fig. 4. (*A*) Chest radiograph showing volume loss and rib cage deformity after multiple left-sided rib fractures. (*B*) Postoperative film at 1 month following metallic strut placement. Note improved volume in the left hemithorax. (*From* Haasler G. Open fixation of flail chest after blunt trauma. Ann Thorac Surg 1990;49:994; with permission. Copyright © 1990, The Society of Thoracic Surgeons.)

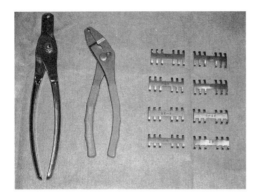

Fig. 5. Judet Struts and application pliers. (*From* Tanaka H, Yukioka T, Yamaguti Y, et al. Surgical stabilization of internal pneumatic stabilization? A prospective randomized study of management of severe flail chest patients. J Trauma 2002;52:729; with permission.)

polymer plates and screws combined with suture cerclage have also been proposed for the management of flail chest (Fig. 8). Plate absorption is believed to result in the gradual transfer of the

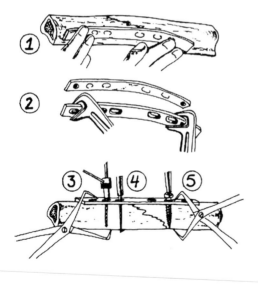
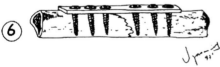

Fig. 6. Schematic of steps 1 through 6 for 3.5-mm acetabular reconstruction plate fixation along each side of the fracture site. (*From* Oyarzun J, Bush A, McCormick JR, et al. Use of 3.5-mm acetabular reconstruction plates for internal fixation of flail chest injuries. Ann Thorac Surg 1998;65:1472; with permission. Copyright © 1998, The Society of Thoracic Surgeons.)

pressure load to the bone, which promotes fracture healing. In addition, the absorbable properties preclude the need for prosthesis extraction [47].

Surgical stabilization can effectively reduce the duration of mechanical ventilatory support and decrease ICU stay. The long-term benefits include restoration of normal chest wall geometry and improved pulmonary function testing. It should be considered in most patients with flail chest who cannot be weaned from the ventilator or have persistent chest pain or chest wall instability despite normal supportive measures. There is no role, however, for surgical stabilization in patients with severe pulmonary contusion. The degree of respiratory failure is a function of the underlying lung injury rather than chest wall motion mechanics.

Summary

Flail chest is an uncommon consequence of blunt trauma. It usually occurs in the setting of a high-speed motor vehicle crash and can carry a high morbidity and mortality. The outcome of flail chest injury is a function of associated injuries. Isolated flail chest may be successfully managed with aggressive pulmonary toilet including facemask oxygen, CPAP, and chest physiotherapy. Adequate analgesia is of paramount importance in patient recovery and may contribute to the return of normal respiratory mechanics. Early intubation and mechanical ventilation is paramount in patients with refractory respiratory failure or other serious traumatic injuries. Prolonged mechanical ventilation is associated with the development of pneumonia and a poor outcome. Tracheotomy and frequent flexible bronchoscopy should be considered to provide effective pulmonary toilet.

Surgical stabilization is associated with a faster ventilator wean, shorter ICU time, less hospital cost, and recovery of pulmonary function in a select group of patients with flail chest. Open fixation is appropriate in patients who are unable to be weaned from the ventilator secondary to the mechanics of flail chest. Persistent pain, severe chest wall instability, and a progressive decline in pulmonary function testing in a patient with flail chest are also indications for surgical stabilization. Open fixation is also indicated for flail chest when thoracotomy is performed for other concomitant injuries. There is no role for surgical stabilization for patients with severe

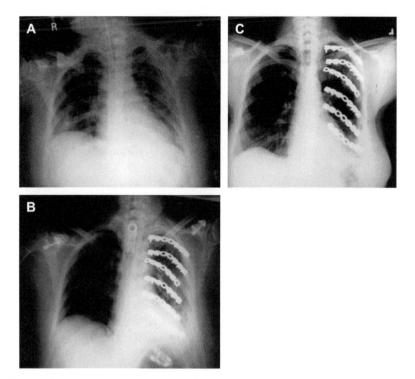

Fig. 7. Chest films made (*A*) preoperatively, (*B*) immediately postoperatively, and (*C*) 1 year postoperatively. (*From* Oyarzun J, Bush A, McCormick JR, et al. Use of 3.5-mm acetabular reconstruction plates for internal fixation of flail chest injuries. Ann Thorac Surg 1998;65:1473; with permission. Copyright © 1998, The Society of Thoracic Surgeons.)

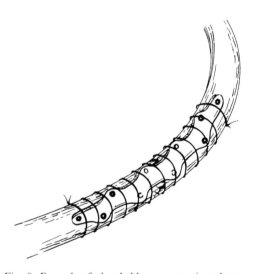

Fig. 8. Example of absorbable reconstruction plate secured with absorbable suture cerclage. (*From* Mayberry J, Terhes J, Ellis T, et al. Absorbable plates for rib fracture repair: preliminary experience. J Trauma 2003;55:836; with permission.)

pulmonary contusion. The underlying lung injury and respiratory failure preclude early ventilator weaning. Supportive therapy and pneumatic stabilization is the recommended approach for this patient subset.

References

[1] National Safety Council 2002. Injury Facts, 2002 edition. Itasca (II): National Safety Council; 2002.

[2] Clark G, Schecter W, Trunkey D. Variables affecting outcome in blunt chest trauma: flail chest vs. pulmonary contusion. J Trauma 1988;28:298–304.

[3] Gaillard M, Herve C, Mandin L, et al. Mortality prognostic factors in chest injury. J Trauma 1990; 30:93.

[4] LoCicero J III, Mattox K. Epidemiology of chest trauma. Surg Clin North Am 1989;69(1):15–9.

[5] Mayberry J, Trunkey D. The fractured rib in chest wall trauma. Chest Surg Clin N Am 1997;7(2): 239–61.

[6] Zuckerman S. Experimental study of blast injuries to the lungs. Lancet 1940;2:219–24.

[7] Viano D, Lau I, Ashbury C. Biomechanics of the human chest, abdomen and pelvis in lateral impact. Accid Anal Prev 1989;21:553–74.

[8] Ciraulo D, Elliott D, Mitchell K, et al. Flail chest as a marker for significant injuries. J Am Coll Surg 1994;178:466–70.

[9] Glinz W. Problems caused by the unstable thoracic wall and by cardiac injury due to blunt injury. Injury 1986;17:322–6.

[10] Miller H, Taylor G, Harrison A, et al. Management of flail chest. Can Med Assoc J 1983;129:1104–7.

[11] Borrelly J, Aazami M. New insights into the pathophysiology of flail segment: the implication of anterior serratus muscle in parietal failure. Eur J Cardiothorac Surg 2005;28:742–9.

[12] Cappello M, Legrand A, De Troyer A. Determinants of rib motion in flail chest. Am J Respir Crit Care Med 1999;159:886–91.

[13] Avery E, Morch E, Benson D. Critically crushed chests: a new method of treatment with continuous mechanical hyperventilation to produce alkalotic apnea and internal pneumatic stabilization. J Thorac Surg 1956;32:291–311.

[14] Cullen P, Modell J, Dirby R. Treatment of flail chest: use of intermittent mandatory ventilation and positive end-expiratory pressure. Arch Surg 1975;110: 1099–103.

[15] Davidson J, Bargh W, Cruickshank A, et al. Crush injuries of the chest: a follow up study of patients treated in an artificial ventilation unit. Thorax 1969;24:563–7.

[16] Duff J, Goldstein M, McLean A, et al. Flail chest: a clinical review and physiological study. J Trauma 1968;8:63–74.

[17] Diethelm A, Battle W. Management of flail chest injury: a review of 75 cases. Am Surg 1971;37:667–70.

[18] Trinkle J, Richardson J, Franz J, et al. Management of flail chest without mechanical ventilation. Ann Thorac Surg 1975;19(4):355–63.

[19] Shanti C, Carlin A, Tyburski J. Incidence of pneumothorax from intercostals nerve block for analgesia in rib fractures. J Trauma 2001;51:536–9.

[20] Mackersie R, Karagianes T, Hoyt DB, et al. Prospective evaluation of epidural and intravenous administration of fentanyl for pain control and restoration of ventilatory function following multiple ribs fractures. J Trauma 1991;31:443–9.

[21] Worthley L. Thoracic epidural in the management of chest trauma: a study of 161 cases. Intensive Care Med 1985;11:312–5.

[22] Dittman M, Ferstl A, Wolff G. Epidural analgesia for the treatment of multiple rib fractures. Eur J Intensive Care Med 1975;1:71–5.

[23] Ward A, Gillatt D. Delayed diagnosis of traumatic rupture of the spleen: a warning of the use of thoracic epidural analgesia in chest trauma. Injury 1989;20:178–9.

[24] Cheema S, Ilsley D, Richardson J, et al. A thermographic study of paravertebral analgesia. Anesthesia 1995;50:18–21.

[25] Karmakar M. Thoracic paravertebral block. Anesthesiology 2001;95:771–80.

[26] Eason M, Wyatt R. Paravertebral thoracic block: a reappraisal. Anesthesia 1979;34:638–42.

[27] Sankaran S, Wilson R. Factors affecting prognosis in patients with flail chest. J Thorac Cardiovasc Surg 1970;60:402–10.

[28] Freedland M, Wilson R, Bender JS, et al. The management of flail chest injury: factors affecting outcome. J Trauma 1990;30(12):1460–8.

[29] Antonelli M, Conti G, Rocco M, et al. A comparison of noninvasive positive pressure ventilation and conventional mechanical ventilation in patients with acute respiratory failure. N Engl J Med 1998;339:429–35.

[30] Hurst J, DeHaven C, Branson R. Use of CPAP mask as the sole mode of ventilatory support in trauma patients with mild to moderate respiratory insufficiency. J Trauma 1985;25:1065–8.

[31] Tanaka H, Tajimi K, Endoh Y, et al. Pneumatic stabilization for flail chest injury: and 11-year study. Surg Today 2001;31:12–7.

[32] Gunduz M, Unlugenc H, Inanoglu K, et al. A comparative study of continuous positive airway pressure (CPAP) and intermittent positive pressure ventilation (IPPV) in patients with flail chest. Emerg Med J 2005;22:325–9.

[33] Voggenreiter G, Neudeck F, Aufmkolk M, et al. Operative chest wall stabilization in flail chest: outcomes of patients with or without pulmonary contusion. J Am Coll Surg 1998;187(2):130–8.

[34] Richardson J, Adams L, Flint L. Selective management of flail chest and pulmonary contusion. Ann Surg 1982;196:481–7.

[35] Kishikawa M, Yoshioka T, Shimazu T, et al. Pulmonary contusion causes long-term respiratory dysfunction with decreased functional residual capacity. J Trauma 1991;31:1203–8.

[36] Johannigman J, Campbell R, Davis K Jr, et al. Combined differential lung ventilation and inhaled nitric oxide therapy in the management of unilateral pulmonary contusion. J Trauma 1997;42:108–11.

[37] Shapiro M, Anderson H, Bartlett R. Resp failure: conventional and high-tech support. Surg Clin North Am 2000;80(3):871–83.

[38] Kause J, Parr M. Extracorporeal membranous oxygenation in the management of severe thoracic trauma: a case report. Crit Care and Resusc 2001; 3(2):97–100.

[39] Voelckel W, Wenzel V, Rieger M, et al. Temporary extracorporeal membranous oxygenation in the treatment of acute traumatic lung injury. Canad J Anesth 1998;45(11):1097–102.

[40] Cacchione R, Richardson D, Seligson D. Painful nonunion of multiple rib fractures managed by operative stabilization. J Trauma 2000;48(2): 319–21.

[41] Lardinois D, Krueger T, Dusmet M, et al. Pulmonary function testing after operative stabilization of the chest wall for flail chest. Eur J Cardiothorac Surg 2001;20:496–501.

[42] Landreneau R, Hinson J, Hazelrigg S, et al. Strut fixation of an extensive flail chest. Ann Thorac Surg 1991;51:473–5.

[43] Tanaka H, Yukioka T, Yamaguti Y, et al. Surgical stabilization of internal pneumatic stabilization? A prospective randomized study of management of severe flail chest patients. J Trauma 2002;52(4):727–32.

[44] Haasler G. Open fixation of flail chest after blunt trauma. Ann Thorac Surg 1990;49:993–5.

[45] Oyarzun J, Bush A, McCormick JR, et al. Use of 3.5-mm acetabular reconstruction plates for internal fixation of flail chest injuries. Ann Thorac Surg 1998;65:1471–4.

[46] Engel C, Krieg J, et al. Operative chest wall fixation with osteosynthesis plates. J Trauma 2005;58:181–6.

[47] Mayberry J, Terhes J, et al. Absorbable plates for rib fracture repair: preliminary experience. J Trauma 2003;55:835–9.

ELSEVIER
SAUNDERS

Thorac Surg Clin 17 (2007) 35–46

THORACIC
SURGERY
CLINICS

Traumatic Injury to the Trachea and Bronchus

Riyad Karmy-Jones, MD[a], Douglas E. Wood, MD[b],*

[a]Heart and Vascular Center, Southwest Washington Medical Center, Suite 300, 200 N.E. Mother Joseph Place,
Vancouver, WA 98664, USA
[b]Division of Cardiothoracic Surgery, University of Washington Medical Center, Box 356310, 1959 NE Pacific Street,
AA-115, Seattle, WA 98195–6310, USA

Tracheobronchial injury is uncommon but immediately life-threatening. The immediate sequelae can include death from asphyxiation, whereas lack of recognition or incorrect management may result in life-threatening or disabling airway stricture. Penetrating injuries can occur with any laceration to the neck or from projectile injuries to the neck or chest. Blunt injuries can occur from a variety of direct and indirect trauma. This article concentrates on injuries that occur between the cricoid cartilage and the right and left mainstem bronchial bifurcations.

Incidence

It is estimated that only 0.5% of all patients with multiple injuries managed in modern trauma centers suffer from tracheobronchial injury [1]. Because virtually all studies of airway trauma combine penetrating and blunt causes and do not publish a denominator of cervical and thoracic injuries with which to calculate the true incidence of airway involvement, however, this is at best a crude estimation.

Penetrating neck injuries have a 3% to 6% incidence of cervical tracheal injury [2]. Less than 1% (4 of 666) of patients admitted with penetrating chest trauma had tracheal injury in a series published from the Ben Taub Hospital in Houston [3]. Based on an annual incidence at major trauma centers of three to four cases of penetrating tracheal trauma per year, it seems that the

incidence of penetrating tracheobronchial trauma constitutes 1% to 2% of thoracic trauma admissions [2,4–6].

Bertelsen and Howitz [7] reviewed 1178 autopsy reports of patients dying of blunt trauma and found an incidence of tracheobronchial injury of 2.8%, with over 80% of these patients dying instantly of airway or associated injuries and the rest dying within 2 hours of reaching the hospital. Kemmerer and associates [8] in 1961 reported an incidence of tracheobronchial rupture of less than 1% in a study of nearly 600 traffic fatalities. Thirty years later, Symbas and colleagues [4] reviewed 20 years of English language literature, spanning from 1970 to 1990, that reported airway injury secondary to blunt trauma. In this time frame, 47 articles described 183 patients, with 6 patients added in the 20-year period from the Grady Memorial Hospital experience in Atlanta.

There has been an apparent increase in the incidence of patients with airway injuries reaching the emergency department alive, which may occur as a result of improved prehospital care and development of specialized regional trauma units [9]. This is difficult to establish, however, given the inherent inaccuracies in the historical and current data regarding airway injuries. De La Rocha and Kayler [10] reported an incidence of tracheobronchial injuries of 1.8% in 327 patients who were discharged from a centralized trauma unit, whereas another series reported an incidence of 0.5% in a series of 2000 patients requiring an intensive care unit admission for multiple trauma [11].

The incidence of tracheobronchial injury seems to be roughly 0.5% to 2% among individuals sustaining blunt trauma, including blunt trauma

---

* Corresponding author.
E-mail address: dewood@u.washington.edu
(D.E. Wood).

1547-4127/07/$ - see front matter © 2007 Elsevier Inc. All rights reserved.
doi:10.1016/j.thorsurg.2007.03.005

to the neck. Most injuries related to blunt trauma involve the intrathoracic trachea and mainstem bronchi. Symbas and coworkers [4] noted the following incidence of injury sites: cervical trachea, 4%; distal thoracic trachea, 22%; right mainstem bronchus, 27%; left proximal mainstem bronchus, 17%; complex injuries involving the trachea and mainstem bronchi, 8%; and lobar orifices, 16%. The rate of tracheobronchial injury from penetrating thoracic trauma is also 0.5% to 2%, but, in contrast, penetrating cervical injuries involve the airway 3% to 8% of the time. Penetrating injuries predominantly involve the cervical trachea, with only 25% of the penetrating injuries involving the intrathoracic airways [2].

Mechanism of injury

Most tracheobronchial injuries result from blunt or penetrating trauma, although iatrogenic injuries and less common causes, such as strangulation, burns, or caustic injury, occasionally result in airway injury. Most penetrating trauma is caused by stab wounds or gunshot wounds and only uncommonly may occur from impalement or slash injuries. Nearly all stab injuries of the trachea are cervical in origin, because of the deep location of the intrathoracic trachea. Knife injuries produce a tearing or shearing effect, resulting in perforation, linear laceration, through-and-through injuries, or transsection [2].

Gunshot wounds are a more common cause of penetrating airway injury and can affect any portion of the cervical or intrathoracic airways. Cervical injuries are still more common, however, being the site of injury in 75% to 80% of penetrating tracheal trauma overall [2]. This may be, in part, because more distal penetrating injuries of the trachea may have associated fatal injuries of the heart or great vessels, and such patients never arrive at the trauma center for evaluation and management. Gunshot wounds produce a crush injury and wound cavity that varies depending on the muzzle velocity, the caliber, and the type of ammunition, with the greatest damage being produced by high-velocity rifles firing hollow-point ammunition. These injuries produce much greater cavitation and soft tissue destruction than do relatively low-velocity injuries from handguns.

Blunt injuries of the cervical trachea most commonly result from direct trauma or from sudden hyperextension. Direct cervical trauma produces a crush injury of the trachea, because it may be impinged on by the rigid vertebral bodies. This has classically been described as a "dashboard" injury because unrestrained automobile passengers may hyperextend the neck during head-on collisions, striking the neck on the steering wheel or dashboard and producing a crush injury of the larynx or cervical trachea [12]. Even the restrained passenger, however, may incur a laryngeal or cervical tracheal injury when a high-riding shoulder harness applies a compressive and rotational force to the neck on front-impact automobile injuries [13]. Clothesline injuries may produce similar direct crushing trauma, but with the force concentrated across a very narrow band. Other injuries may occur with rapid hyperextension, producing a traction and distraction injury that most commonly results in laryngotracheal separation. Hyperextension injuries most commonly occur in automobile crashes, but can occur in any other situations in which forced rapid cervical hyperextension occurs.

Kirsh and associates [14] proposed three potential mechanisms for the cause of blunt intrathoracic tracheobronchial injuries. First, they noted that sudden, forceful anteroposterior compression of the thoracic cage is the most common type of injury associated with tracheobronchial disruption. They postulated that this produces a decrease in the anteroposterior diameter with subsequent widening of the transverse diameter. Because the lung remains in contact with the chest wall because of negative intrapleural pressure, lateral motion pulls the two lungs apart, producing traction on the trachea at the carina. Airway disruption occurs if this lateral force exceeds tracheobronchial elasticity. A second mechanism may be caused by airway rupture as a consequence of high airway pressures. Compression of the lung, trachea, and major bronchi between the sternum and vertebral column during blunt trauma produces a sudden increase in intratracheal airway pressure; and in a patient with a closed glottis at the moment of impact, rupture can occur when the intraluminal pressure exceeds the elasticity of the membranous trachea and bronchi. Rupture in these circumstances occurs most commonly at the junction of the membranous and cartilaginous airway or between cartilaginous rings. The third potential mechanism may be caused by a rapid deceleration injury, producing shear forces at points of relative airway fixation, such as the cricoid cartilage and the carina, similar to the mechanism of traumatic injuries of the thoracic aorta.

Associated injuries

Because of the adjacent cervical and intrathoracic structures, penetrating airway trauma frequently is associated with significant associated injuries that often are major determinants of outcome. Blunt trauma is often associated with multiple injuries involving not only chest, but abdomen, head, and orthopedic structures [15]. Cervical trauma of the airway frequently involves the esophagus, the recurrent laryngeal nerves, the cervical spine and spinal cord, the larynx, and the carotid arteries and jugular veins. Intrathoracic penetrating trauma may involve the esophagus, left recurrent laryngeal nerve, and spinal cord, but it can also involve any of the great vessels, including the ascending arch and descending aorta and the pulmonary arteries, and may involve any of the four heart chambers or the lung parenchyma. Obviously, concomitant great vessel and cardiac injury from penetrating trauma is frequently fatal and may lead to exsanguination or asphyxiation of blood in the airway before presentation in a trauma unit. These associated injuries are common and frequently determine the ultimate outcome in terms of the patient's survival and morbidity.

Kelly and colleagues [16] reported on a series of 100 penetrating tracheobronchial injuries. Among patients with injury in the cervical trachea, 28% had an associated esophageal injury, 24% had a hemopneumothorax, 13% had a major vascular injury, 8% had a recurrent laryngeal nerve injury, and 3% had a spinal cord injury. In contrast, primary injuries of the intrathoracic trachea were associated with an incidence of esophageal injury of 11%; hemopneumothorax, 32%; a major vascular injury, 18%; cardiac injury, 5%; spinal cord injury, 7%; and intra-abdominal injuries, 18%. Several other series have shown an overall incidence of associated major injuries with penetrating tracheobronchial trauma to be in the range of 50% to 80%, most of these being esophageal and vascular injuries, followed by spinal cord, pulmonary, and intra-abdominal injuries [4–6,17,18].

Because of the magnitude of blunt trauma necessary to produce an airway injury, associated injuries are also common in this group and may be the primary determinant in patient outcome. Any other structure or organ system may be involved as in any multiple trauma patient. Head, facial, and cervical spine injuries are frequent and important predictors of mortality and morbidity.

Blunt intra-abdominal, intrathoracic, and skeletal trauma also occurs frequently, as do specific injuries to the esophagus and great vessels that are adjacent to the major airways. Major associated injuries are present in 40% to 100% of patients suffering blunt airway trauma and are dominated by orthopedic injuries in most patients, with a third to half of the patients having concomitant facial trauma, pulmonary contusions, or intra-abdominal injuries. Ten percent to 20% of the patients have major closed-head injuries, and approximately 10% have associated spinal cord injuries [15,18]. In one series, a very high incidence was reported of recurrent nerve injury associated with blunt airway trauma as evidenced by vocal cord dysfunction without evidence of direct laryngeal injury [19]. In this series, 49% of patients had recurrent nerve injuries and two thirds of these had bilateral recurrent nerve palsy. In this same series, a 21% incidence of esophageal perforation was reported, clearly suggesting the need for high index of suspicion for associated esophageal injuries, even in the setting of blunt trauma. A high percentage of cervical crush injuries producing tracheal disruption may have associated laryngeal injuries that require careful assessment by an otolaryngologist during the primary assessment phase and before treatment decisions are made regarding repair of the tracheal injury.

Diagnosis

Airway injuries become the first priority in trauma, and because of their acuity and critical importance in stabilizing the patient, initial steps in management may proceed simultaneously with the diagnosis of airway pathology and associated injuries. Dyspnea and respiratory distress are frequent symptoms, occurring in 76% to 100% of patients [16,18,19]. The other common symptom is hoarseness or dysphonia, which occurred in 46% of the patients in a series published by Reece and Shatney [19].

The most common signs of airway injury reported in most series were subcutaneous emphysema (35%–85%); pneumothorax (20%–50%); and hemoptysis (14%–25%) [16,18–21]. Air escaping from a penetrating wound in the neck is a pathognomonic sign of airway laceration and occurs in approximately 60% of patients with cervical penetrating trauma to the trachea [5]. A cervical air leak that ceases after intubation confirms the diagnosis.

The most useful initial diagnostic studies are those obtained routinely in the initial trauma survey (ie, chest and cervical spine radiographs). Deep cervical emphysema and pneumomediastinum are seen in 60% and pneumothorax occurs in 70% of patients with tracheobronchial injuries [21,22]. The cervical spine or chest radiograph may also show a disruption of the tracheal or bronchial air column on careful examination. Overdistention of the endotracheal tube balloon cuff or displacement of the endotracheal tube may give additional radiologic signs of airway injury [22]. Complete transsection of a mainstem bronchus may result in the classic signs of atelectasis; "absent hilum"; or a collapsing of the lung away from the hilus toward the diaphragm, known as the "falling lung sign of Kumpe" (Fig. 1) [23–25]. A persistent pneumothorax with large air leak from a well-placed chest tube should increase the suspicion of intrathoracic tracheal or bronchial injury. With the chest tube on suction, the patient may experience more respiratory difficulties, and this finding is almost invariably associated with bronchial disruption [26].

Although neck and upper chest CT scan has become critical to the accurate diagnosis of traumatic laryngeal injuries, the role in more distal tracheobronchial injuries is not well established [12]. Commonly, a chest CT may be obtained as a part of the trauma work-up and is extremely valuable in detecting the presence of

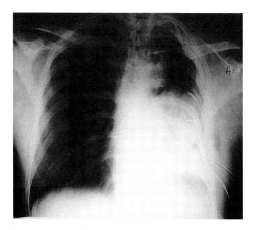

Fig. 1. Chest radiograph of a patient following blunt trauma. The patient presents with persistent left-sided pneumothorax and collapsed lung despite tube thoracostomy without air leak. The lung has collapsed down with the hemi-thorax because of complete separation of the left main stem bronchus.

a mediastinal hematoma or the possibility of associated injuries of the great vessels. The CT scan may show mediastinal air, disruption of the tracheobronchial air column, deviation of the airway, or the specific site of airway disruption (Fig. 2). Although not specifically indicated for the work-up of suggested acute tracheobronchial trauma, preoperative CT can be useful in assessing associated laryngeal injuries or other unsuspected chest injuries that should be dealt with at the time of surgical exploration. CT is contraindicated in the hemodynamically unstable trauma patient or the patient with an unstable airway. A negative CT scan does not obviate the need for bronchoscopy or other diagnostic studies. CT bronchography, or virtual bronchoscopy, may be helpful in some cases [27]. Experience suggests that this is best when a CT is done for other reasons, and there is suspicion of injury rather than performing CT primarily with the view of obtaining a CT bronchogram.

Other imaging of suspected associated injuries is performed as indicated. Because of the common association of esophageal injuries, particularly after penetrating trauma, a contrast esophagogram is often necessary. Esophageal injuries may be distant from the airway injuries because of the distortion of tissues on traumatic impact [28]. Angiography (either intra-arterial or CT angiography) of the aortic arch or cervical vessels is performed for penetrating injuries in a stable patient or in a blunt chest trauma patient when the chest radiograph raises the suspicion for great vessel injury or aortic injury.

If the initial diagnosis of airway injury is missed, granulation tissue and stricture of the trachea or bronchus develops within the first 1 to 4 weeks and usually leads to symptoms, signs, and radiologic findings of pneumonia, bronchiectasis, atelectasis, and abscess. Stridor and dyspnea are the common signs of late tracheal stenosis, whereas wheezing and postobstructive pneumonia are the common presentations of bronchial stenosis. Chest radiography and CT have been useful in the delayed setting and may directly reveal the site of stenosis and the secondary consequences of airway narrowing.

Bronchoscopy provides the single definitive diagnostic study in a patient with suspected airway injury. Direct or fiberoptic laryngoscopy is an important part of the endoscopic study in patients with cervical trauma and should be performed with the assistance of an experienced otolaryngologist when laryngeal injuries are

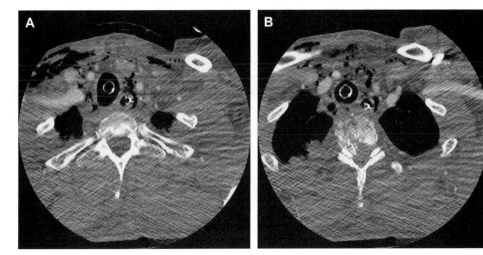

Fig. 2. (A, B) Neck CT arteriogram of a patient with a gunshot wound to the neck. There is extensive subcutaneous emphysema but no clear area of tracheal or esophageal injury discernible from the imaging. The arteriogram is important to exclude underlying penetrating vascular trauma before surgical exploration of the trachea and esophagus.

suggested. Careful examination of the tracheobronchial tree with the fiberoptic bronchoscope allows determination of the site and extent of injury. Bronchoscopy is the only study that can reliably exclude central airway trauma, although minor lacerations may occasionally be missed. The advantages of fiberoptic bronchoscopy are that it can be performed quickly and easily, even in the setting of concomitant head and neck injuries or cervical spine trauma. If bronchoscopy is being performed for a suspected airway injury in an intubated patient, it is important carefully to withdraw the endotracheal tube during endoscopy to avoid missing proximal tracheal injuries.

Initial airway management

The initial and most important priority in acute tracheobronchial injury is to secure a satisfactory airway. Patients with respiratory distress and the clinical suspicion of an airway injury should be intubated immediately, preferably with the guidance of a flexible bronchoscope, as described previously. If the patient is unstable either hemodynamically or in terms of respiratory status, however, the optimal first method still remains oral entubation with in-line cervical stabilization.

In a stable patient, fiberoptic intubation provides several advantages. First, it does not require neck extension for direct laryngoscopy and so can

be performed while stabilization of the cervical spine is maintained before the exclusion of cervical spine injuries. Second, fiberoptic intubation can easily be performed in the awake, spontaneously ventilating patient. This prevents the need for sedation and paralysis, which is contraindicated in the patient with an unstable airway, until a satisfactory airway can be established. Sedation and paralysis is also contraindicated during the immediate evaluation and stabilization of an injured patient who requires several simultaneous assessments and hemodynamic stabilization. Third, flexible bronchoscopy can act as an obturator for the endotracheal tube and direct the tube past an area of injury under direct vision, allowing accurate placement into the distal trachea or either mainstem bronchus as necessary. Lastly, immediate bronchoscopy by an experienced endoscopist allows early evaluation of the location and extent of airway injury. This provides the best early information about the indications and approach for airway repair, allowing this to be calculated into the priority list of possible interventions for the multiply injured patient.

In published reports, the incidence of upper airway obstruction or severe distress that requires immediate intubation is variable and dependent on the degree of injuries and the criteria used. Flynn and associates [21] reported 8 (36%) of 22 patients requiring an immediate airway, and 3 of these patients requiring an emergency tracheostomy or cricothyroidotomy. A series by Gussack and colleagues [1] revealed 92% of patients requiring an emergency airway, 73% of these being successfully managed by orotracheal intubation and three emergently intubated through an open neck wound. Edwards and associates [29] and Rossbach and coworkers [18] reported that approximately 60% of their patients required prompt control of the airway. In Rossbach and Johnson's series, 74% of the patients requiring emergency intubation were successfully managed by orotracheal intubation alone, whereas 10% required intubation with fiberoptic guidance, 10% were intubated through an open neck wound, and only one patient (5%) required an emergent surgical airway through tracheostomy or cricothyroidotomy [18]. In the series reported by Edwards and coworkers [29], approximately 60% of the emergency airways were managed by nasotracheal or orotracheal intubation, and the other 40% required tracheostomy. Important points are raised concerning the three patients in this series who were initially stable but experienced sudden deterioration secondary to the airway injury while they were being evaluated for multiple injuries. Two patients with a transsected cervical trachea required emergency tracheostomy with intubation of the distal tracheal segment through the tracheostomy incision. In one patient, an attempted emergency cricothyroidotomy produced a significant laryngeal injury that necessitated subsequent delayed repair [29]. A high index of suspicion and prompt securing of the injured airway are paramount to both the initial resuscitation and the ultimate outcome.

Patients with air emanating from a penetrating cervical injury may be intubated through the neck injury directly into the tracheal lumen. This technique has been used in approximately 25% of airway trauma in reports that include penetrating cervical injuries [1,18,21,29]. Attempts at oral intubation or blind intubation through a cervical wound may be futile, however, and can either precipitate total obstruction or allow the progressive loss of an unstable airway if repeated attempts are unsuccessful. Although intubation guided by a flexible bronchoscope may solve most of these difficulties, delay in obtaining a bronchoscope or successfully traversing the injury may also cause complete obstruction, with the tragic loss of a salvageable patient. In cases in which airway injury is suspected, preparation for immediate tracheostomy must be made simultaneously with the attempts at intubation. In cases of severe maxillofacial trauma, immediate

tracheostomy is the procedure of choice for airway control. Cricothyroidotomy is rarely useful in tracheobronchial trauma because the injury lies distal to the insertion point of the tracheostomy tube, which is placed blindly and with no additional accuracy over oral or nasotracheal intubation alone. If a tracheostomy is performed, the tracheostomy tube should be placed through the area of injury if possible to prevent extension of the tracheal injury by the tracheal stoma. A transsected cervical trachea may retract into the mediastinum; in these cases, it is best found by inserting a finger into the mediastinum anterior to the esophagus, locating the distal trachea by palpation, and grasping the clamp to allow retraction into the cervical wound and distal intubation [30].

Management of the airway for injuries of the distal trachea, the carina, and the proximal mainstem bronchi can be extremely challenging. Use of double-lumen tubes should be avoided because of their rigidity and size, which increases the possibility of injury extension. In these cases, a long endotracheal tube should be positioned beyond the injury or into the appropriate mainstem bronchus to provide single-lung ventilation. This can best be performed with the aid of the flexible bronchoscope serving as a guide and to confirm the final position. In almost all cases, standard ventilation can be initiated once distal airway control is ensured. In cases of distal injuries of the left mainstem bronchus, the bronchus intermedius, or lobar orifices, a bronchial blocker placed proximal to the injury under endoscopic guidance provides another alternative for stabilizing the airway and allowing ventilation.

Anesthetic management

Close cooperation between the anesthesiologist and surgeon is critical to the successful management of a tracheobronchial injury. In most cases a long, single-lumen tube is not only sufficient, but safe. In selected circumstances, use of an endobronchial blocker or carefully passed double lumen tube may be required.

In hemodynamically stable patients, high-frequency jet ventilation provides an effective option for ventilation with relatively low airway pressures. Its main advantage is during airway reconstruction, because it can be delivered through a small catheter with less bulk and rigidity, allowing easier placement of sutures or approximation of the newly reconstructed airway without tension. In most cases, however, it is usually easiest to perform standard ventilation through the oral endotracheal tube or through a sterile endotracheal tube inserted through the operative field into the transsected airway. This does not require additional equipment or experience and has the added advantage of a cuffed tube preventing aspiration of blood into the distal airway and less aerosolization of blood around the surgical team.

Cardiopulmonary bypass is virtually never necessary for the intraoperative management of isolated airway injuries. Associated injuries of the heart or great vessels may require cardiopulmonary bypass. In cases in which cardiopulmonary bypass is already being used, it may facilitate a concomitant tracheobronchial repair. Cardiopulmonary bypass after major trauma can exacerbate intracerebral or intra-abdominal hemorrhage, however, and potentiate the systemic inflammatory response that produces adult respiratory distress syndrome, with a very high subsequent mortality. In simple injuries, standard ventilation is straightforward, precluding consideration of cardiopulmonary bypass. In complex injuries, or those in which associated trauma makes ventilation difficult, the anticoagulation and added trauma of cardiopulmonary bypass probably results in exacerbation of bleeding and the systemic inflammatory response more than it helps in allowing airway repair.

Virtually all patients with isolated tracheobronchial injuries can be easily extubated at the end of the operative procedure and should be managed by the anesthesiologist with this in mind. Patients who require postoperative ventilation because of their associated injuries should finish the procedure with a large-bore, single-lumen endotracheal tube to allow good pulmonary toilet and fiberoptic bronchoscopy if necessary. If possible, this should be placed with the balloon cuff distal to the area of tracheal repair in proximal injuries or should lie proximal and away from the repair for carinal and mainstem bronchial injuries. Major laryngeal or maxillofacial injuries with the anticipated need for prolonged ventilation are indications for placement of a tracheostomy at the completion of the tracheobronchial repair. This tracheostomy should not be placed through the tracheal repair, which leads to a contamination of the suture line with subsequent dehiscence or stenosis [30].

Surgical management

Minor injuries may not be initially apparent or recognized, because of a lack of clinical suspicion or concealment by prompt distal intubation for stabilization of a patient with multiple injuries. These minor injuries may heal without direct surgical repair without negative sequelae if they involve less than one third of the circumference of the airway. Mucosal defects, not associated with ongoing air leak, may also heal and do not require immediate intervention. The most reliable short- and long-term result is provided by prompt, definitive repair, however, and should be performed whenever possible when the injury is recognized. In rare circumstances it may be appropriate to perform a delayed repair if it is not possible to perform operative correction because of the instability of the patient with multiple injuries.

The proximal one half to two third of the trachea is best approached through a low cervical collar incision that also provides excellent exposure to vascular or esophageal injuries in the neck. Creating a "T" incision over the manubrium and splitting the manubrium down to the second interspace opens the thoracic inlet and provides a broader exposure to the middle third of the trachea and proximal control of the innominate artery or veins. A full median sternotomy does not provide significant additional airway exposure except in specific circumstances, which are discussed later. The distal third of the trachea, the carina, and the right mainstem bronchus are most easily approached through a right thoracotomy, which also provides good exposure to the azygous vein, superior vena cava, and right atrium, and most of the intrathoracic esophagus. Injuries of the left mainstem bronchus are most easily approached through a left thoracotomy, which also provides good exposure to the distal portion of the aortic arch, the descending thoracic aorta, and the proximal left subclavian artery. Exposure to the proximal left mainstem, the carina, the distal trachea, or the right mainstem is extremely difficult through a left thoracotomy, however, because of the overlying aortic arch. Adequate proximal exposure may be gained by mobilization of the arch with retraction cephalad and laterally and division of the ligamentum arteriosum.

These approaches may not be adequate for the management of potential associated injuries. Because of the proximity of the heart and great vessels anterior to the distal trachea, the carina, and the proximal mainstem bronchi, penetrating injuries to the chest are likely to have associated life-threatening cardiovascular injuries. A median sternotomy is often performed to provide optimal access to the heart or great vessels but provides far less satisfactory exposure to the trachea, carina, and bronchi than the respective thoracotomies. It is possible, however, to obtain exposure to the anterior airway in the vicinity of the carina to allow anterior repair or limited primary resection and reconstruction. This requires mobilization of the superior vena cava with reflection to the right, retraction of the ascending aorta to the left, and longitudinal division of the posterior pericardium cephalad to the right pulmonary artery and caudal to the innominate vein. Unfortunately, this does not provide any exposure to the posterior airway where blunt injuries frequently occur. It also does not provide adequate exposure for repair of concomitant esophageal injuries. A bilateral thoracosternotomy or "clamshell" incision through the fourth interspace provides good exposure to both hemithoraces and the anterior mediastinum and may be considered as an approach because of associated injuries. This approach provides little additional airway exposure or airway advantages, however, over those incisions previously described.

Simple, clean lacerations without airway devascularization can be repaired primarily with simple interrupted absorbable sutures. The authors prefer 4-0 Vicryl (Ethicon, Cincinnati, Ohio), although others have successfully used permanent and absorbable monofilament. Simple longitudinal disruption of the membrane away from its junction with the rings can be managed by resuspending the membrane with interrupted sutures. In cases in which there is significant tracheobronchial damage, all devitalized tissue should be débrided, with care taken to preserve as much viable airway as possible. In these cases, a circumferential resection and end-to-end anastomosis is almost always preferable to partial wedge resections of traumatized airway with attempted primary repair. The principles of airway resection and reconstruction are similar for tracheal, carinal, or bronchial injuries, although the anatomy of reconstruction is unique to the surgical exposure, the location, and the extent of resection. This is particularly true when a portion of the carina must be resected or reconstructed, because a large variety of techniques may be necessary to achieve reconstruction in this area [31]. Dissection of the airway is limited to the region to be resected to preserve tracheobronchial blood supply to the area of anastomosis. Precise placement of interrupted absorbable suture allows an airtight anastomosis, correction of size discrepancy between the distal and proximal airway, and minimal anastomotic granulations if the anastomosis is brought together without tension.

In most patients, up to half of the trachea can be resected and primarily reconstructed, so that the most significant tracheal injuries should be able to allow primary resection and reconstruction without difficulty. Both mainstem bronchi can be completely resected with primary reconstruction without tension in all cases. Extensive injuries of the carina are more problematic and should be repaired rather than resected if at all possible. Only 3 to 4 cm of airway involving the carina can be resected and allow for primary reconstruction. A variety of tracheobronchial release maneuvers have been used to allow a tension-free anastomosis. For most limited tracheal resections, blunt development of the anterior avascular pretracheal plane combined with neck flexion is all that is necessary. For more extensive proximal tracheal resections, a suprahyoid laryngeal release can provide 1 to 2 cm of additional proximal mobilization. For resections of the mainstem bronchi or carina, division of the pericardium around the inferior aspect of the hilum provides an additional 1 to 2 cm of distal airway mobilization [32].

Associated injuries of the esophagus should be repaired in two layers. When working through an anterior cervical exposure, the esophagus may be best exposed by complete tracheal transsection through the area of planned tracheal repair. A vascularized flap of muscle or soft tissue should be interposed between the tracheal and esophageal repairs to minimize the risk of postoperative tracheoesophageal fistula. Intrathoracic tracheobronchial suture lines are also preferably wrapped with pedicled pericardial fat, intercostal muscle, or pleura to separate the airway anastomosis from overlying blood vessels. In cases in which a portion of the trachea or carina has been resected and reconstructed, much of the airway mobility is provided by neck flexion. This position is maintained in the postoperative period by placement of a "guardian suture" between the chin and the sternum. Patients with isolated airway injuries are routinely extubated in the operating room, even after complex reconstructions.

Postoperative management

Careful airway observation is maintained in the early postoperative period. Aggressive pulmonary toilet, including the liberal use of bedside bronchoscopy, is important because these patients may have difficulty clearing secretions past their anastomosis or area of airway repair. Patients who have an associated vocal cord paralysis may have even more difficulty with pulmonary toilet because of their inability to produce an effective cough. These patients may benefit from a commercially available mini tracheostomy (Minitrach II, Portex, Keene, New Hampshire), which is placed through their cricothyroid membrane to allow direct tracheal suctioning. Some patients with tracheal resection may have problems with postoperative aspiration because of difficulty in elevating the larynx during deglutition. This is more profound in the patients with associated recurrent nerve injuries or in those who have had a suprahyoid laryngeal release. The remainder of the postoperative management is similar to the routine care after other neck operations or thoracotomy for pulmonary resection. In the trauma setting, management of the associated injuries and their complications may dominate the care of the patient. For the ventilated patient, care should be taken to position the endotracheal balloon distal or proximal to the tracheal suture line and minimize airway pressures in cases where the endotracheal tube lies above the airway anastomosis by necessity. These patients should be managed at the lowest possible airway pressures that provide satisfactory oxygenation and ventilation and extubated as soon as their other injuries allow. Bronchoscopy should usually be performed 7 to 10 days after tracheobronchial repair or before discharge to ensure satisfactory healing without granulation tissue or the early development of anastomotic stenosis.

Complications

The complications of tracheobronchial repair are similar to those of airway resection and reconstruction and consist mostly of anastomotic problems. Anastomotic dehiscence or restenosis occurs in 5% to 6% of patients after tracheal reconstruction [33]. Initial management involves securing the airway, usually with an endoluminal or tracheal T tube until healing is complete and the perioperative inflammation has subsided. Most of these patients can be managed with subsequent airway resection and reconstruction 3 to 6 months after the original repair if necessary [34,35]. Anastomotic dehiscence is life-threatening if this results in fistula formation to the innominate artery or esophagus. Tracheal and innominate artery fistula is rare but frequently fatal and requires immediate operation for division of the innominate artery and interposition of healthy tissue between the airway and great vessels. Tracheoesophageal fistula can usually be managed initially by establishing gastric drainage, enteral nutrition, and treatment of pneumonia. When the patient is stable and no longer requires ventilatory support, the tracheoesophageal fistula can be divided, with the esophageal and tracheal defects resected or repaired and healthy soft tissue interposed between the adjacent suture lines. If vocal cord paralysis is permanent, it can usually be palliated by vocal cord lateralization or medialization procedures.

Late presentation

Patients may incur delayed treatment after tracheobronchial trauma for three reasons. First, the initial injury may have been subtle and initially missed in the early or intermediate trauma management. Second, severe associated injuries may have prevented early definitive management of recognized airway injury. Third, initial attempts at repair may fail, resulting in dehiscence or late stenosis.

In any of these scenarios, the sequelae are similar. Although the airway may be partially or completely disrupted at the time of initial injury, it may be held together by strong peritracheal connective tissue, allowing an airway to be established and ventilation to be maintained. As the primary injury or secondary dehiscence heals, however, granulation tissue and scar contracture result, with subsequent stricture formation that usually develops 1 to 4 weeks after injury. Taskinen and associates [36] reported nine patients with blunt tracheobronchial rupture, five of whom had operations purposely delayed from 9 to 89 days because of complete lung expansion with suction drainage. In all five patients, however, dyspnea later developed, with bronchoscopy revealing obstruction and granulation tissue at the site of airway injury. Each of these patients required subsequent airway resection with primary reconstruction.

These patients may initially have dyspnea on exertion but may also have wheezing, stridor, cough, difficulty in clearing secretions, or recurrent respiratory infections. Any of these symptoms with a history of trauma or prolonged intubation should raise the suspicion of a late airway stenosis, which should be diagnosed or excluded by bronchoscopy. A 50% reduction in the cross-sectional area of the trachea usually results in dyspnea only with significant exertion, whereas narrowing of the lumen to less than 25% usually produces dyspnea and stridor at rest. Patients may be reasonably compensated despite significant stenosis but can have acute life-threatening deterioration with a minor amount of airway edema or secretions. A high index of suspicion in these patients is critical to their subsequent work-up and timely diagnosis [9].

Once recognized, critical airway stenosis can be evaluated and initially stabilized by bronchoscopy and dilatation [37]. The appropriate, definitive management of most of these patients is subsequent tracheal or bronchial resection with primary reconstruction as for benign airway strictures from other causes. Except in cases of distal lung destruction by chronic infection, re-establishment of ventilation to lung parenchyma can be expected to restore significant function, even years after the injury. There may be little or no apparent function by preoperative perfusion scanning; this is likely caused by reflexive pulmonary vasoconstriction and is reversible on resumption of ventilation to the lung parenchyma. Airway reconstruction should always be considered first in these instances, with pulmonary resection reserved for patients with unreconstructable lesions or those with destroyed parenchyma from chronic infection or bronchiectasis.

Results

Injury to the trachea and proximal bronchi is a lethal injury, with more than 75% of patients with blunt tracheobronchial trauma dying before arrival to the emergency department [7]. There are no known series of autopsy studies of penetrating tracheobronchial trauma to give a similar prehospital mortality denominator. In both instances, however, death is most likely caused by associated injuries rather than by the tracheobronchial injury itself.

In patients operated on for penetrating injuries, the mortality is 6% to 18% [5,6]. Of 17 survivors of penetrating tracheal trauma, 88% had a good result, apparently without symptoms [6]. One of 17 patients had permanent hoarseness from concomitant recurrent nerve injury and a second patient required a permanent tracheostomy

because of complications and failed reconstruction of a combined tracheal and esophageal injury. In Rossbach's and coworkers [18] series of 32 patients with penetrating (59%) and blunt (41%) tracheobronchial trauma, 78% of patients required postoperative mechanical ventilation. In patients with a penetrating injury, this ranged from 1 to 3 days with a mean of 2 days, and in patients with blunt injury, intubation ranged from 3 to 9 days with a mean of 5 days. The average length of intensive care unit stay was 4 days for patients with penetrating trauma and 9 days for patients with blunt injury, whereas the mean hospitalization was 15 days and 17 days for penetrating and blunt injuries, respectively. Nineteen percent of patients in this series sustained postoperative complications, but 93% of patients were ultimately asymptomatic and returned to preinjury function. Only 1 (3%) of 32 patients had a symptomatic late stenosis after repair of complex avulsion injury. The mortality rate in this series was 6% and was related to multiple injuries in the setting of blunt trauma. Results from other series show a mortality of 10% to 25% for patients undergoing repair of tracheobronchial injury in the setting of penetrating or blunt trauma with associated injuries [4,21,29].

Patients with early definitive airway repair had a long-term good result in over 90% of patients, with poor airway–related outcomes generally being caused by associated recurrent nerve injury or failed initial tracheobronchial repair [1,19]. In the series by Reece and Shatney [19], however, good results were only obtained in 67% of patients who had tracheal repair over a stent or with a tracheostomy, leaving the authors to conclude that primary early repair provides the best long-term outcomes. In many series, the ultimate prognosis after airway injury is dependent on the associated injuries, particularly closed-head injuries. Thirteen percent of the patients in a series published by Angood and associates [11] were left in a vegetative state, despite excellent functional airways, after definitive tracheobronchial repair.

Summary

Tracheobronchial injuries are relatively uncommon, often require a degree of clinical suspicion to make the diagnosis, and usually require immediate management. The primary initial goals are twofold: stabilize the airway and define the extent and location of injury. These are often facilitated by flexible bronchoscopy, in the hands of a surgeon capable of managing these injuries. Most penetrating injuries occur in the cervical area. Most blunt injuries occur in the distal trachea or right mainstem, and are best approached by a right posterolateral thoracotomy. Choice and timing of approach are dictated by the presence and severity of associated injuries. The mainstay of intraoperative management remains a single-lumen endotracheal tube. Most injuries can be repaired by simple techniques, using interrupted sutures, but some require complex reconstructive techniques. Follow-up to detect stenosis or anastomotic technique is important, as is attention to pulmonary toilet.

References

[1] Gussack GS, Jurkovich GJ, Luterman A. Laryngotracheal trauma: a protocol approach to a rare injury. Laryngoscope 1986;96:660–5.

[2] Lee RB. Traumatic injury of the cervicothoracic trachea and major bronchi. Chest Surg Clin N Am 1997;7:285–304.

[3] Graham JM, Mattox KL, Beall AC Jr. Penetrating trauma of the lung. J Trauma 1979;19:665–9.

[4] Symbas PN, Justicz AG, Ricketts RR. Rupture of the airways from blunt trauma: treatment of complex injuries. Ann Thorac Surg 1992;54:177–83.

[5] Symbas PN, Hatcher CR Jr, Vlasis SE. Bullet wounds of the trachea. J Thorac Cardiovasc Surg 1982;83:235–8.

[6] Symbas PN, Hatcher CR Jr, Boehm GA. Acute penetrating tracheal trauma. Ann Thorac Surg 1976;22:473–7.

[7] Bertelsen S, Howitz P. Injuries of the trachea and bronchi. Thorax 1972;27:188–94.

[8] Kemmerer WT, Eckert WG, Gathright JB, et al. Patterns of thoracic injuries in fatal traffic accidents. J Trauma 1961;1:595–9.

[9] Karmy-Jones R, Jurkovich GJ. Blunt chest trauma. Curr Probl Surg 2004;41:211–380.

[10] de la Rocha AG, Kayler D. Traumatic rupture of the tracheobronchial tree. Can J Surg 1985;28:68–71.

[11] Angood PB, Attia EL, Brown RA, et al. Extrinsic civilian trauma to the larynx and cervical trachea: important predictors of long-term morbidity. J Trauma 1986;26:869–73.

[12] Lupetin AR. Computed tomographic evaluation of laryngotracheal trauma. Curr Probl Diagn Radiol 1997;26:185–206.

[13] Guertler AT. Blunt laryngeal trauma associated with shoulder harness use. Ann Emerg Med 1988; 17:838–9.

[14] Kirsh MM, Orringer MB, Behrendt DM, et al. Management of tracheobronchial disruption secondary to nonpenetrating trauma. Ann Thorac Surg 1976; 22:93–101.

[15] Ramzy AI, Rodriguez A, Turney SZ. Management of major tracheobronchial ruptures in patients with multiple system trauma. J Trauma 1988;28:1353–7.

[16] Kelly JP, Webb WR, Moulder PV, et al. Management of airway trauma. I: tracheobronchial injuries. Ann Thorac Surg 1985;40:551–5.

[17] Grover FL, Ellestad C, Arom KV, et al. Diagnosis and management of major tracheobronchial injuries. Ann Thorac Surg 1979;28:384–91.

[18] Rossbach MM, Johnson SB, Gomez MA, et al. Management of major tracheobronchial injuries: a 28-year experience. Ann Thorac Surg 1998;65: 182–6.

[19] Reece GP, Shatney CH. Blunt injuries of the cervical trachea: review of 51 patients. South Med J 1988;81: 1542–8.

[20] Baumgartner F, Sheppard B, de Virgilio C, et al. Tracheal and main bronchial disruptions after blunt chest trauma: presentation and management. Ann Thorac Surg 1990;50:569–74.

[21] Flynn AE, Thomas AN, Schecter WP. Acute tracheobronchial injury. J Trauma 1989;29:1326–30.

[22] Stark P. Imaging of tracheobronchial injuries. J Thorac Imaging 1995;10:206–19.

[23] Endress C, Guyot DR, Engels JA. The "fallen lung with absent hilum" signs of complete bronchial transection. Ann Emerg Med 1991;20:317–8.

[24] Kumpe DA, Oh KS, Wyman SM. A characteristic pulmonary finding in unilateral complete bronchial transection. Am J Roentgenol Radium Ther Nucl Med 1970;110:704–6.

[25] Wintermark M, Schnyder P, Wicky S. Blunt traumatic rupture of a mainstem bronchus: spiral CT demonstration of the "fallen lung" sign. Eur Radiol 2001;11:409–11.

[26] Deslauriers J, Beaulieu M, Archambault G, et al. Diagnosis and long-term follow-up of major bronchial disruptions due to nonpenetrating trauma. Ann Thorac Surg 1982;33:32–9.

[27] Jones CM, Athanasiou T. Is virtual bronchoscopy an efficient diagnostic tool for the thoracic surgeon? Ann Thorac Surg 2005;79:365–74.

[28] Minard G, Kudsk KA, Croce MA, et al. Laryngotracheal trauma. Am Surg 1992;58:181–7.

[29] Edwards WH Jr, Morris JA Jr, DeLozier JB III, et al. Airway injuries: the first priority in trauma. Am Surg 1987;53:192–7.

[30] Mathisen DJ, Grillo H. Laryngotracheal trauma. Ann Thorac Surg 1987;43:254–62.

[31] Mitchell JD, Mathisen DJ, Wright CD, et al. Clinical experience with carinal resection. J Thorac Cardiovasc Surg 1999;117:39–52 [discussion: 52–3].

[32] Heitmiller RF. Tracheal release maneuvers. Chest Surg Clin N Am 2003;13:201–10.

[33] Grillo HC, Zannini P, Michelassi F. Complications of tracheal reconstruction: incidence, treatment,

and prevention. J Thorac Cardiovasc Surg 1986;91: 322–8.

[34] Wright CD, Grillo HC, Wain JC, et al. Anastomotic complications after tracheal resection: prognostic factors and management. J Thorac Cardiovasc Surg 2004;128:731–9.

[35] Donahue DM, Grillo HC, Wain JC, et al. Reoperative tracheal resection and reconstruction for unsuccessful repair of postintubation stenosis.

J Thorac Cardiovasc Surg 1997;114:934–8 [discussion: 938–9].

[36] Taskinen SO, Salo JA, Halttunen PE, et al. Tracheobronchial rupture due to blunt chest trauma: a follow-up study. Ann Thorac Surg 1989;48: 846–9.

[37] Stephens KEJ, Wood DE. Bronchoscopic management of central airway obstruction. J Thorac Cardiovasc Surg 2000;119:473–7.

THORACIC
SURGERY
CLINICS

Thorac Surg Clin 17 (2007) 47–55

Hemothorax Related to Trauma

Dan M. Meyer, MD

Department of Thoracic and Cardiovascular Surgery, University of Texas Southwestern
Medical Center at Dallas, 5323 Harry Hines Boulevard, Dallas, TX 75390–8879, USA

The most common cause of hemothorax is trauma. In 1794, John Hunter first advocated incision and drainage of hemothoraces through the intercostal space. This was in contrast to the common view at the time that conservative management was the correct treatment. Although Hunter's method of evacuation of the hemothorax was effective, the pneumothorax required to explore the chest added significant morbidity. By the 1870s, however, evacuation of hemothoraces with trochars or catheters was becoming standard therapy.

Much of the experience with management of thoracic injuries related to either empyema or pneumothorax. Using many variations on the same theme, Van Swieten [1] recommended evacuating traumatic hemothorax through a blunt-tipped flexible tube perforated laterally with suction applied. Baudens [2], a military surgeon, in 1830, used a rubber urethral catheter and a bulb syringe to evacuate a traumatic hemothorax from a gunshot wound but placed the catheter into the soft tissue, not the thoracic cavity. Playfair [3] introduced waterseal drainage of a chest tube in 1875. Importantly, Graham's [4] work during World War I with closed drainage of the chest led to adoption of this technique during World War II for the management of more thoracic trauma [5]. Although closed tube thoracostomy drainage of the thorax following thoracotomy was first reported by Lilienthal in 1922 [6], this system for traumatic hemothorax was not used widely until the Korean War.

Demographics

Chest trauma is the most common cause of traumatic death in the United States after head trauma, accounting for about 20% of deaths [7]. Blunt trauma from motor vehicle crashes has accounted for 70% to 80% of thoracic injuries [8]. In a study representative of the typical urban trauma experience, 1359 consecutive chest trauma patients presenting to a Level 1 trauma center in the United States were reviewed. Surprisingly, only 18% of patients required tube thoracostomy, and only 2.6% required thoracotomy [9]. As is typical of the trauma population, the patients were predominantly male (70.9%), with 48% of the individuals belonging to the 20- to 49-year-old group. A total of 90% of the injuries were from a blunt mechanism. Associated trauma included long bone injuries, which occurred in 28% of patients. The liver (8.5%) and the spleen (7.4%) were the most commonly sited injuries in the abdominal cavity. A low Glasgow Coma Scale and advanced age were the most significant independent predictors of mortality. The overall mortality in this study was 9.4% (128 patients) with the cause of death being noncardiothoracic in approximately 37%. Moreover, 56% of deaths occurred within the first 24 hours.

Blunt chest wall injuries may cause a hemothorax, but the trauma to the underlying lung is usually of greater consequence. Rib fractures may be the culprit, causing bleeding from an intercostal vessel or associated pulmonary parenchymal injury as the source of the hemorrhage. More significant hemothoraces from blunt injuries may be secondary to a major injury, such as an intrathoracic vascular structure. In a study of 1490 blunt chest trauma patients, Liman and associates [10] found a significant correlation

E-mail address: dan.meyer@utsouthwestern.edu

between the number of rib fractures and mortality. The overall mortality rate was 1%, 4.7% in patients with more than two rib fractures, and 17% for those with flail chest. The patients' age and Injury Severity Score also were significantly related to mortality rate. The rate of development of pneumothorax or hemothorax was 6.7% in patients with no rib fracture, 24.9% in patients with one or two rib fractures, and 81.4% in patients with more than two rib factures. Tube thoracostomy was required in 260 patients, or 17.4% of their patients. Standard surgical intervention was required in only 12 patients in their series. Overall, these authors concluded that the risk of mortality was associated with the presence of more than two rib fractures, with patients over the age of 60 years and with an Injury Severity Score greater than or equal to 16 in chest trauma.

Penetrating chest trauma clearly causes direct injury to a chest wall vessel, and equally common is injury to the lung or heart itself. Moreover, injuries of the vascular tree could also be the source, but usually these are processes not simply managed with tube thoracostomy.

Diagnostic assessment

Physical examination

The use of physical examination to detect hemothoraces in chest trauma patients is often questioned, because all patients with significant chest trauma receive radiographic imaging. Bokhari and colleagues [11] studied 676 trauma patients to determine in which patient population physical examination could have more benefit than chest radiograph (CXR). In their series of 523 blunt chest trauma patients, the negative predictive values of auscultation and pain or tenderness were 100% and 99%. The sensitivity of auscultation and pain or tenderness was 100% and 57%. In contrast, in 153 penetrating chest trauma patients, the negative predictive values were less than 91%, with sensitivities of auscultation, pain or tenderness, and tachypnea 50%, 25%, and 32%, respectively. They concluded that blunt chest trauma patients who are hemodynamically stable with a normal physical examination may not require a routine CXR. In contrast, all patients suffering penetrating trauma require chest radiographs to detect hemopneumothorax in the absence of clinical findings. Although all patients presenting to the emergency department with chest trauma likely get a CXR, confidence in the accuracy of the physical examination may allow necessary intervention before waiting for the CXR.

Focused assessment with sonography for trauma

Access to ultrasonography in the emergency department, now considered the standard of care, incorporates views of both pleural spaces and confirms a clinical suspicion of hemothorax and allows for early intervention before radiographic identification. Any pleural effusion is visible above the diaphragm as an anechoic space, and this may indicate the presence of a traumatic hemothorax (Fig. 1). As the name implies, focused assessment with sonography for trauma (FAST) returns data more quickly than standard radiography (1.3 versus 14.2 minutes) [12]. In a prospective study of 61 trauma patients, Brooks and associates [13] demonstrated ultrasonography to have a sensitivity of 92%, a specificity of 100%, a positive predictive value of 100%, and a negative predictive value of 98%. Ultrasound results were compared with the finding on either CXR, the presence of blood drained from the chest, and occasionally as chest CT scan. In 84% of the cases, the ultrasound results were available to the trauma team before the plain radiographs. These results, however, are in contrast to a study by Abboud and Kendall [14] that demonstrated a lower sensitivity (12.5%) and an acceptable specificity (98.4%).

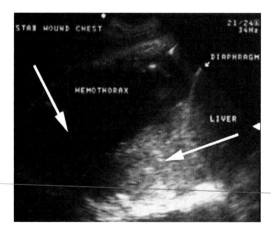

Fig. 1. Emergency department focused assessment with sonography for trauma image of a hemothorax seen above the right diaphragm from a stab wound. Shown are an anechoic area of nonclotted blood (*left arrow*) and echoic clotted blood (*right arrow*).

Chest radiograph

Bleeding into the pleural space may originate from injury to the pleura, chest wall, lung, diaphragm, or mediastinum. An upright CXR is the standard initial and primary diagnostic study in the evaluation of hemothoraces (Fig. 2). The presence of any blunting of the costophrenic angle equates to approximately 200 mL of blood that may be present in the pleural space. As the volume of fluid increases, a meniscus sign may be seen. This is in contrast to a hemopneumothorax, with which an air-fluid level is demonstrated. A supine CXR allows layering of the hemothorax in the dependent, posterior portion of the pleural space. In this situation, a vague opacification of one hemothorax relative to the other may be appreciated, with up to 1000 mL of blood potentially present in the pleural space of these patients. As the hemothorax increases in size, compression of the lung parenchyma may be visualized. A large hemothorax may also cause mediastinal shift away from the side of the injury.

Chest CT

High-resolution, spiral CT technology has enabled the detection of even small hemothoraces.

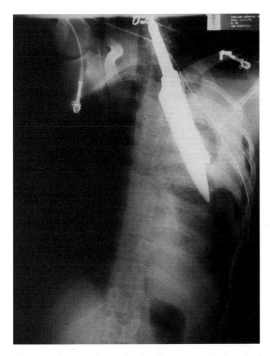

Fig. 2. Chest radiograph showing a retained apical hemothorax after a penetrating injury to the left chest.

In the acute trauma setting, the presence of fluid is blood unless proved otherwise. In the subacute situation, however, more uncommon possibilities exist. In these cases, an appreciation of the Hounsfield units may help categorize the fluid. A measurement of 35 to 70 HU may represent a hemothorax, whereas a sympathetic serous effusion, which may be associated with significant intra-abdominal process, may have a measurement of less than 15 HU (Fig. 3).

Thoracentesis

Diagnostic thoracentesis is not typically used in the acute trauma setting. Rarely, in the subacute period, characterization of a fluid collection could be clarified by the use of thoracentesis. This diagnostic tool has no role in the acute trauma setting. Even more uncommonly, the diagnosis of chylothorax, from trauma to the thoracic duct, or the rare bilious effusion could be detected by thoracentesis.

Management

Tube thoracostomy

Most chest trauma can be managed without thoracotomy. Well-positioned tube thoracostomies and more recently thoracoscopy has limited the need for formal thoracotomy. Although there have been advocates in the past to allow the stable hemothorax to resolve spontaneously, there remains a risk of empyema and fibrothorax that is better managed by prevention. Regarding

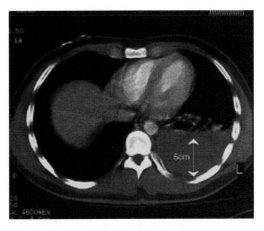

Fig. 3. CT scan depicting a large hemothorax with fluid collection (>4.5 cm lamellar fluid stripe) in the dependent pleural gutter on transverse axial image.

placement of the thoracostomy tube, a 32F or 36F catheter is recommended, with positioning in the mid- to posterior axillary line tracking posteriorly. Furthermore, placement low in the thoracic cage (sixth or seventh intercostal space) provides optimal drainage. In situations where the post-tube thoracoscostomy CXR demonstrates incomplete drainage, options include placement of another drainage tube or thoracoscopic exploration and drainage.

Use of video-assisted thoracic surgery

Before the acceptance and experience with thoracoscopic techniques, placement of a second chest tube was the standard management for the retained hemothorax. When this was unsuccessful, thoracotomy soon followed. To assess the use of thoracoscopy in the setting of traumatic hemothoraces, a randomized prospective study was performed comparing the use of an additional chest tube versus thoracoscopy in this population (Fig. 4) [15]. Results showed that patients undergoing thoracoscopy had a shorter duration of chest tube drainage compared with those patients who had an additional CT placed (2.53 ± 1.36 versus 4.50 ± 2.83 days; $P < .02$). The duration of hospital stay was also diminished in the group undergoing thoracoscopy (5.40 ± 2.16 versus 8.13 ± 4.62 days; $P < .02$). Hospital costs were also significantly less in the thoracoscopy group ($7689 + $3278 versus $13,273 + $8158 days; $P < .02$). There was no mortality in either group. The authors concluded that early intervention with video-assisted thoracoscopic surgery (VATS) may be a more efficient and economic strategy for managing retrained hemothoraces after trauma (Table 1).

More recently, Navsaria and associates [16] reviewed their experience with 46 patients with retained hemothoraces after penetrating trauma.

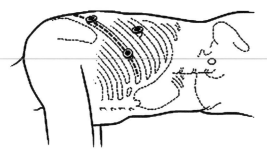

Fig. 4. Patient positioning and thoracoscopic port placement for potential conversion to thoracotomy.

They reported an 80% success rate of thoracoscopy for evacuation of the clotted hemothorax, whereas in 20%, conversion to open thoracotomy was required. In these patients, there were significant adhesions that inhibited the ability fully to explore and evacuate the hemothorax thoracoscopically. Surprisingly, the failure of VATS did not correlate with the median time elapsed from injury to surgery: 12 days for thoracotomy versus 10 days for thoracoscopy ($P = .139$). A strategy that more rapidly addresses the retained hemothorax as was demonstrated in the prior trial [15], specifically directly after the first tube thoracostomy is found to be ineffective, should allow for more successful management of this problem.

Thoracotomy

Indications for acute intervention because of massive hemothorax have been fairly standard and include drainage of at least 1500 mL blood with initial chest tube placement, more than 200 mL/h for 4 hours, or a combination of these values in the face of hemodynamic instability. In the acute setting, left or right posterolateral thoracotomies are not tolerated hemodynamically and not recommended. Sternotomy offers the most options for suspected injuries to the heart or great vessels. Moreover, in injuries at or above the sternal angle, sternotomy is again recommended as the primary approach. For penetrating injuries to the left of the left mid-clavicular line and below the level of the sternal angle, a left anterior thoracotomy approach is also appropriate. For suspected injuries to the right of the right parasternal line, however, median sternotomy is also recommended, because in the acute setting there is no role for right anterior thoracotomy. In the subacute setting, lateral or posterolateral thoracotomies offer better access to the area that may require exploration at the time of hemothorax evacuation.

In a study addressing the issue of early thoracotomy for trauma, Karmy-Jones and colleagues [17] reviewed 157 patients who underwent urgent thoracotomy (defined as surgery within 48 hours of injury because of persistent bleeding) in five major urban trauma centers. Most patients suffered penetrating trauma. They found three general indications for thoracotomy in this setting: (1) shock or cardiopulmonary arrest with suspected correctable intrathoracic lesion; (2) specific diagnoses (eg, penetrating cardiac or blunt aortic injury); and (3) evidence of persistent

Table 1
Comparison of clinical outcomes between patient groups based on initial randomization strategy

Intent to treat	Duration of tube drainage (d)	Hospital days after the procedure	Total hospital days	Estimated costs ($)
Group 1	4.50 ± 2.83	7.21 ± 5.30[a]	8.13 ± 4.62[a]	13,273 ± 8158
Group 2	2.53 ± 1.36	3.60 ± 1.64	5.40 ± 2.16	7689 ± 3278

Results are presented as mean ± standard deviation.
[a] $P < .02$ by Student t test.

thoracic hemorrhage, defined as persistent bleeding after an initial chest tube output of at least 1500 mL or a continued hourly blood loss greater than 250 mL for 3 consecutive hours after tube thoracostomy. They found mortality rate increased as the total chest blood loss increased, with the risk for death at a blood loss of 1500 mL being three times greater than at 500 mL. The absolute amount of blood loss, rather than the hourly output, may be the more important value to emphasize.

Patients with blunt thoracic trauma were associated with a significantly worse prognosis than for penetrating injury. Much of this increased mortality is related to the increased confounding factors after blunt injury, such as pulmonary contusion, abdominal injury, or pelvic fracture. In situations where a large output of blood is obtained initially from the chest tube, but the patient remains hemodynamically stable and there is no further evidence of hemorrhage, thoracotomy is usually not indicated. With this exception, Karmy-Jones and associates [17] concluded that persistent thoracic hemorrhage, although a more common indication for thoracotomy after penetrating injury, is not unusual after blunt trauma. Thoracic bleeding of greater than 1500 mL within the first 24 hours of admission after injury is a simpler criterion to prompt consideration of performing thoracotomy.

Management of occult traumatic hemothoraces

With the liberal use of CT scanning in evaluating trauma patients, hemothoraces that are not typically considered significant on CXR may be visualized on either the chest or abdominal CT scans. A retrospective study by Bilello and colleagues [18] of 78 patients with occult hemothoraces assessed the lamellar fluid stripe in the dependent pleural gutter on transverse axial cuts. Those patients with a lamellae less than 1.5 cm were considered minimal, whereas those with

at least 1.5 cm of fluid were termed "moderate-large" effusion. Patients with a hemothorax of at least 1.5 cm of fluid were four times more likely to undergo drainage (8 patients in the minimal group, 31 patients in the moderate-large group) intervention compared with those having hemothorax less than 1.5 cm.

Thrombolytic infusion

Oguzkaya and associates [19] reviewed their experience with thoracoscopy versus intrapleural streptokinase for the management of posttraumatic retained hemothoraces. Over a 10-year period, 31 cases were managed by intrapleural streptokinase (250,000 U/100 mL saline/24 h) and 34 patients by videothoracoscopy. Although there were no deaths in either group, the use of videothoracoscopy was significantly better than instillation of intrapleural streptokinase both in terms of the need for thoracotomy (nine cases versus two cases; $P < .02$) and duration of hospital stay (14.5 ± 4.2 days versus 9.8 ± 3.7 days; $P < .0001$).

Late complications of hemothoraces

Late complications of the retained hemothorax include empyema and fibrothorax. Empyema is the result of bacterial contamination of the residual hemothorax, which can result in bacteremia and generalized sepsis. Fibrothorax, conversely, is problematic but not immediately life-threatening. The effect of the organized clot on the visceral pleural, however, can lead to incomplete expansion of the lung and direct effects on pulmonary function.

Empyema

In an extensive review of empyema after trauma, Mandal and colleagues [20] reported the incidence of this complication in 5474 patients over a 24-year period. The incidence of empyema was 1.6%, with empyema being defined by radiographic findings of a persistent and loculated pleural fluid collection, a fever greater than 380°C, with leukocytosis ($>12,000$ cells/mm^3), or with a septic course that could not be explained by any other process than the one noted in the thorax. Most patients (91%) were cured without the need for thoracotomy. Instead, they depended on tube thoracostomy or image-guided catheter drainage. The time course of the study (1972–1996) predated most experience with VATS for this indication. More recent experience with VATS for posttraumatic empyema has been promising [21]. The inciting organism was most commonly *Staphylococcus aureus*, followed by anaerobic bacteria. Because of the need to treat large numbers of patients to prevent a single empyema and the emergence of resistant organisms, the authors believed that presumptive antibiotic therapy was contraindicated in the management of chest trauma patients with tube thoracostomies because antibiotic therapy does not reduce the incidence of empyema or pneumonia in these patients. Because of the overall low incidence of empyema in the trauma population, they did not recommend prophylactic antibiotics for trauma patients requiring tube thoracostomy.

In a review of patients with blunt thoracic trauma, Watkins and associates [22] assessed the frequency of empyema and restrictive pleural processes and described how this contributed to the patients' degree of respiratory failure. Although the CXRs in these patients were generally nondiscriminating, the CT scans showed previously unrecognized fluid collections, air-fluid levels, or gas bubbles. Neither thoracentesis nor placement of additional chest tubes was helpful. Moreover, positive cultures were uncommon. The authors believed that CT imaging has become a very valuable tool in aiding their diagnosis of empyema in complex, critically ill patients. The investigators also noted that the excellent response of their patients to thoracotomy and decortication suggested that empyema was a major factor in the pathogenesis of their respiratory failure and ventilator

dependence. Watkins and associates [22] believe that pleural space infections may cause or contribute to the development of respiratory failure in up to 10% of patients after blunt trauma. Nevertheless, Watkins and associates [22] emphasized that open thoracotomy and decortication has produced excellent results in similar patients in many centers including their own. Because of the morbidity related to thoracotomy and decortication (39% suffered significant complications), however, a more aggressive approach has been made toward early thoracoscopic exploration and evacuation [23].

The use of presumptive antibiotics in tube thoracostomy

The most recent attempt at assessing the use of presumptive antibiotics in patients requiring tube thoracostomy for traumatic hemothoraces comes from a multicenter study of 224 patients [24]. In this prospective, randomized, double-blind trial comparing the use of cefazolin, it was found that the duration of tube placement and thoracic acute injury score were predictive of empyema ($P<.05$) (Table 2). As seen in the table, patients in group A received antibiotics throughout the duration of the chest tube placement, Group B only continued the antibiotics for 12 to 24 hours after the incident, and Group C advocated being a control group. Presumptive antibiotic use did not significantly affect the incidence of empyema or pneumonia, although no empyema occurred in the group that received antibiotics. The authors note that there have been seven reports in the literature demonstrating favorable results with antibiotic therapy in the management of chest tubes for trauma, and three studies have indicated no therapeutic benefit from presumptive antibiotics.

To develop evidence-based guidelines for prophylactic (preventive) antibiotic use for trauma patients requiring a chest tube, Luchette,

Table 2
Incidence of empyema and pneumonia by study group and by mechanism of injury

Study Group	Empyema			Pneumonia		
	Blunt (%)	Penetrating (%)	Total (%)	Blunt (%)	Penetrating (%)	Total (%)
Group A (N = 77)	0	0	0	5 (6.4)	1 (1.3)	6 (7.8)
Group B (N = 76)	1 (0.4)	1 (0.4)	2 (2.5)	6 (7.9)	0	6 (7.8)
Group C (N = 71)	2 (0.9)	2 (0.9)	4 (5.6)	2 (2.8)	0	2 (2.8)
Total (N = 224)	3 (1.3)	3 (1.3)	6 (2.6)	13 (5.8)	1 (0.4)	14 (6.3)

Pasquale, and the other members of the EAST Practice Management Guidelines Work Group [25] used 11 articles identified to formulate the guidelines for prophylactic antibiotic use in trauma patients with a tube thoracostomy. The data in this evidentiary table are listed alphabetically by class and include four class I articles, five class II, and two class III meta-analyses. They concluded that sufficient class I and II data were provided by these 11 articles to recommend prophylactic antibiotic use in patients receiving tube thoracostomy after penetrating or blunt chest trauma. A first-generation cephalosporin should be administered for no longer than 24 hours. These data suggest that this may reduce the incidence of pneumonia but not empyema in trauma patients with tube thoracostomy. Multiple factors were believed to contribute to the development of post-traumatic empyema in chest-trauma patients undergoing tube thoracostomy and included (1) the conditions whereby the tube is inserted (emergent or urgent); (2) the mechanism of injury; (3) retained hemothorax; and (4) ventilator care. The administration of antibiotics for longer than 24 hours did not seem significantly to reduce this risk compared with a shorter duration, although the numbers of patients in each series were small.

Controversies

Sequencing of operative procedures in thoracoabdominal injuries

Selecting the more critical area of concern, the abdomen or the chest in patients with thoracoabdominal injuries is often an area of controversy between trauma and thoracic surgeons. In the age of selective short-term delay of thoracic aortic repair, most studies have favored stabilization, and operative management of abdominal injuries if necessary before thoracotomy. Even in 1982, when the study by Borman and associates [26] was presented, they found the sequence of first operating on the abdominal injury, then the chest, as being not only safe but necessary for optimal survival. More recently, Asensio and colleagues [27] reviewed a broader group of thoracoabdominal trauma patients and found that inappropriate sequencing of the procedures occurred in 44% of patients undergoing combined procedures. Determining whether the missile trajectory has crossed the diaphragm to involve an adjacent cavity is often difficult, however, and rarely completely accurate or predictable. If the wrong cavity is explored

first, additional risk and possibly death may be the price imposed. Clearly, the two critical decisions that must be made first when evaluating these patients are which body cavity must be accessed first and the precise timing.

The authors found the most frequent causes of inappropriate sequencing of laparotomy and thoracotomy in patients with thoracoabdominal injures were persistent unexplained hypotension unaccounted for by the surgical findings in the initial cavity accessed, and misleading chest tube output, both of which were considered indications that the wrong body cavity had been accessed initially. Other important pitfalls included the need to access another body cavity for exposure or mobilization of the liver, and injuries missed during the early evaluation that later manifested during the intraoperative course.

The authors point out that opening another body cavity to exclude injury (ie, quick thoracotomy or laparotomy) should not be practiced indiscriminately or routinely. The physiologic implications can be devastating and may promote hypothermia and its sequelae, increase the operating time in severely compromised patients, and place the patient at risk for iatrogenic injury. Penetrating thoracoabdominal injuries incurred a 31% mortality rate, which increased to 59% for the 73 patients requiring combined thoracotomy and laparotomy. This doubled mortality rate was because of the inappropriate sequencing of the laparotomies and thoracotomies, which occurred in 32 (44%) of 73 patients undergoing combined procedures.

Emergency department thoracotomy

In a comprehensive effort by the Ad Hoc Subcommittee on Outcomes of the American College of Surgeons—Committee on Trauma, Ascencio and members of the Working Group published Practice Management Guidelines for Emergency Department Thoracotomy [28]. Although the indications for performing emergency department thoracotomy have been quite varied over the years, outcomes of patients treated for penetrating cardiac injuries have been acceptable. Of the recorded total of 1165 patients receiving emergency department thoracotomy for penetrating injury, 31% of the patients survived. Although some series have selected outcomes-oriented physiologic parameters, only three studies have statistically validated their predictive values. Most of these series omit data pertaining to the physiologic status of the patient on initial presentation.

Issues to be considered in assessing patients for resuscitative emergency department thoracotomy include the mechanism of injury of the potential patient; the prospectively validated physiologic predictors of outcomes, if any, that can safely and accurately identify patients who will benefit from the procedure and also safely exclude those who will not; the true survival rates of this procedure; and the incidence of severe neurologic impairment in those patients who do survive. Following evidenced-based medicine guidelines, the Working Group, Ad Hoc Subcommittee on Outcomes of the American College of Surgeons—Committee on Trauma recommended the following.

Level I

There is insufficient evidence to support a Level I recommendation for this practice guideline. This topic does not lend itself to be studied with prospective randomized controlled trials.

Level II

1. Emergency department thoracotomy should rarely be performed in patients sustaining cardiopulmonary arrest secondary to blunt trauma because of its very low survival rate and poor neurologic outcomes. Emergency department thoracotomy should be limited to those who arrive with vital signs at the trauma center and have a witnessed cardiopulmonary arrest.
2. Emergency department thoracotomy is best applied to patients sustaining penetrating cardiac injuries who arrive at trauma centers after a short time at the scene of the injury and rapid transport time to the trauma center where they have a witnessed cardiopulmonary arrest or have objectively measured physiologic parameters (ie, signs of life) including pupillary response, spontaneous ventilation, presence of carotid pulse, measurable or palpable blood pressure, extremity movement, and cardiac electrical activity.
3. Emergency department thoracotomy should be performed in patients sustaining penetrating noncardiac thoracic injuries, but these patients generally have a low survival rate. Because it is difficult to ascertain whether the injuries are noncardiac thoracic versus cardiac, emergency department thoracotomy can be used to establish the diagnosis.
4. Emergency department thoracotomy should be performed in patients sustaining exsanguinating abdominal vascular injuries, although these patients generally have a low survival rate. Judicious selection of patients should be exercised. This procedure should be used as an adjunct to definitive repair of the abdominal-vascular injury.

Summary

Management of hemothoraces related to trauma follows basic tenets well-respected by both trauma and cardiothoracic surgeons. In most, a nonoperative approach is adequate with a defined group of patients requiring only tube thoracostomy. It is only in a true minority of individuals that operative intervention is necessary. In blunt thoracic injuries, the underlying organ damage may be the more life-threatening process, not the presence or absence of a hemothorax. For both blunt and penetrating injuries, the presence of retained hemothorax is well-treated by early intervention with thoracoscopic techniques, shown to decrease hospital stay and costs. Controversial areas including the use of prophylactic antibiotics, sequence of operative intervention in patients with combined thoracoabdominal trauma, and the use of emergency department thoracotomy, remain a challenge but recent literature can serve to guide the clinician.

References

[1] Van Swieten G. Boerhaave: aphorisms. London: W and J Innys; 1724. p. 75–8.
[2] Baudens ML. Clinique des Plaies d'Armes a Few. Paris: Bailliere; 1886. p. 289–90.
[3] Playfair GE. Case of empyema treated by aspiration and subsequently by drainage: recovery. Br Med J 1875;1:45.
[4] Graham EA. A brief account of the development of thoracic surgery and some of its consequences. Surg Gynecol Obstet 1957;104:241.
[5] Berry FB. Early treatment of chest wounds by intrapleural suction. Bull U S Army Med Dep 1948;8:211.
[6] Lilienthal H. Pulmonary resection for bronchiectasis. Ann Surg 1922;75:257.
[7] LoCicero J, Mattox KL. Epidemiology of chest trauma. Surg Clin North Am 1989;69:15–9.
[8] Shorr RM, Crittendenn M, Indeck M, et al. Blunt thoracic trauma: analysis of 515 patients. Ann Surg 1987;206:200–5.

[9] Kulshrestha P, Munshi I, Wait R. Profile of chest trauma in a level I trauma center. J Trauma 2004; 57:576–81.

[10] Liman ST, Kuzucu A, Irfan A, et al. Chest injury due to blunt trauma. Eur J Cardiothorac Surg 2003;23: 374–8.

[11] Bokhari F, Brakenridge S, Nagy K, et al. Prospective evaluation of the sensitivity of physical examination in chest trauma. J Trauma 2002;53:1135–8.

[12] Sisley AC, Rozycki GS, Ballard RB, et al. Rapid detection of traumatic effusion using surgeon-performed ultrasonography. J Trauma 1998;44: 291–6.

[13] Brooks A, Davies B, Sethhurst M, et al. Emergency ultrasound in the acute assessment of haemothorax. Emerg Med J 2004;21:44–6.

[14] Abboud PC, Kendall J. Emergency department ultrasound for hemothorax after blunt traumatic injury. J Emerg Med 2003;25(2):181–4.

[15] Meyer DM, Jessen ME, Wait MA, et al. Early evacuation of traumatic retained hemothoraces using thoracoscopy: a prospective, randomized trial. Ann Thorac Surg 1997;64(5):1396–400.

[16] Navsaria PH, Vogel RJ, Nicol AJ. Thoracoscopic evacuation of retained posttraumatic hemothorax. Ann Thorac Surg 2004;78:282–6.

[17] Karmy-Jones R, Jurkovich GJ, Nathens AB, et al. Timing of urgent thoracotomy for hemorrhage after trauma: a multicenter study. Arch Surg 2001;136: 513–8.

[18] Bilello JF, Davis JW, Lemaster DM. Occult traumatic hemothorax: when can sleeping dogs lie? Am J Surg 2005;190:844–8.

[19] Oguzkaya F, Ackah Y, Bilgin M. Videothoracoscopy versus intrapleural streptokinase for management of post traumatic retained haemothorax: a retrospective study of 65 cases. Injury, Int J Care Injured 2005;36:526–9.

[20] Mandal AK, Thadepalli H, Mandal AK, et al. Posttraumatic empyema thoracis: a 24-year experience at a major trauma center. J Trauma 1997; 43(5):764–71.

[21] Landrenau RJ, Keenan RJ, Hazelrigg SR, et al. Thoracoscopy for empyema and hemothorax. Chest 1995;109:18.

[22] Watkins JA, Spain DA, Richardson D, et al. Empyema and restrictive pleural processes after blunt trauma: an under-recognized cause of respiratory failure. Am Surg 2000;66:210–4.

[23] Heniford BT, Carrillo EH, Spain DA, et al. The role of thoracoscopy in the management of retained thoracic collections after trauma. Ann Thorac Surg 1997;63:940–3.

[24] Maxwell RA, Campbell DJ, Fabian TC, et al. Use of presumptive antibiotics following tube thoracostomy for traumatic hemopneumothorax in the prevention of empyema and pneumonia: a multicenter trial. J Trauma 2004;57(4):742–9.

[25] Lukette FA, Barrie PS, Oswanski MF, et al. Practice management guidelines for prophylactic antibiotic use in tube thoracoscopy for traumatic hemopneumothorax: The EAST practice management guideline working group. J Trauma 2000;484:753–7.

[26] Borman KR, Aurbakken CM, Weigelt JA. Treatment priorities in combined blunt abdominal and aortic trauma. Am J Surg 1982;144:728–32.

[27] Asensio JA, Arroyo H Jr, Veloz W, et al. Penetrating thoracoabdominal injuries: ongoing dilemma— which cavity and when? World J Surg 2002;26: 539–43.

[28] Asensio J, Wall M, Minei J, et al. Practice management guidelines for emergency department thoracotomy. Working Group, Ad Hoc Subcommittee on Outcomes, American College of Surgeons-Committee on Trauma. J Am Coll Surg 2001; 193(3):303–9.

ELSEVIER
SAUNDERS

Thorac Surg Clin 17 (2007) 57–61

THORACIC
SURGERY
CLINICS

Blunt Traumatic Lung Injuries

Daniel L. Miller, MD[a],*, Kamal A. Mansour, MD[b]

[a]Section of General Thoracic Surgery, Department of Surgery, Emory University and The Emory Clinic,
1365 Clifton Road NE, Atlanta, GA 30322, USA
[b]Emory University School of Medicine, 1365 Clifton Road NE, Atlanta, GA 30322, USA

The first detailed description of chest trauma appeared in the Edwin Smith Papyrus in ancient Egypt circa 1600 BC [1]. In the fifth century BC, Hippocrates described hemoptysis after rib fractures. He recognized that hemoptysis indicated injury to the underlying lung, which was a more severe injury than a simple rib fracture [2]. Approximately one third of all patients admitted to major trauma centers in the United States sustain serious injuries to the chest. The lungs, which occupy a large portion of the chest cavity and lie in close proximity to the bony thorax, are injured in the majority of these patients directly or indirectly. A significant number of lung injuries are also associated with trauma to other critical thoracic structures. This article discusses blunt trauma injuries of the lung, which include pulmonary contusions, hematomas, lacerations, and pulmonary vascular injuries.

Pulmonary contusion

Pulmonary contusion is the most common injury seen in association with thoracic trauma [3]. It occurs in 30% to 75% of patients sustaining major chest injuries [4]. Pulmonary contusion is seen with blunt and penetrating wounds but is most common after motor vehicle accidents when the chest strikes the steering wheel or car door. The incidence of pulmonary contusions may be decreasing because of supplementary restraint systems, known as airbags, installed in US automobiles. Air bags supplement the safety

belt by reducing the chance that the occupant's upper body will strike the vehicle's interior. They also help reduce the risk of serious injury by distributing crash forces more evenly across the occupant's body. This decrease in lung injuries has been evident at Grady Memorial Hospital in Atlanta, Georgia, one of the busiest level I trauma centers in the United States. From January 1, 2001 through December 31, 2006, a total of 8780 patients were admitted to the Emory University Trauma Service; 989 patients (11%) had an associated lung injury related to their trauma. Pulmonary contusions can also occur after falls from great heights or from blast injuries.

Isolated pulmonary contusions are encountered much less commonly than are contusions associated with other thoracic and nonthoracic injuries. Because pulmonary contusions are so commonly associated with other injuries, the pathophysiology of the associated injuries, the resuscitative and therapeutic measures that are necessary for their treatment, and the effects of aspiration, infection, and adult respiratory distress syndrome (ARDS) on the lung parenchyma have clouded the understanding of isolated pulmonary contusion.

Pathology

Wagner and colleagues [5] presented convincing evidence based on CT scan findings and limited pathologic material that a pulmonary laceration with resultant hemorrhage into adjacent alveolar spaces, rather than alveolar capillary wall injury, is the basis for the development of pulmonary contusions. They described four types of lacerations that are associated with pulmonary contusions. Type I lacerations are the result of compression

---

* Corresponding author.
   E-mail address: daniel.miller@emoryhealthcare.org (D.L. Miller).

1547-4127/07/$ - see front matter © 2007 Published by Elsevier Inc.
doi:10.1016/j.thorsurg.2007.03.017

thoracic.theclinics.com

of the elastic chest wall that causes the underlying air-filled lung to rupture. Type II lacerations result from compression of the lower chest wall that causes a sudden displacement of the lower lobe across the vertebral column and that produces a shearing tear in the adjacent lung. Type III lacerations are small peripheral lacerations that are close to rib fractures and are thought to be penetrating injuries caused by the ends of the fractured ribs. Type IV lacerations are tears caused by sudden chest wall compression that displaces the lung inwardly next to thick pleuropulmonary adhesions. Type I is the most commonly encountered laceration and is almost always seen in patients who are younger than 40 years of age. Type III lacerations are the next most commonly seen and usually occur in older patients.

Diagnosis

Blunt trauma to the chest, falls, and blast injuries should all suggest the possibility that a pulmonary contusion may occur. Dyspnea, tachypnea, hemoptysis, cyanosis, and hypotension are frequently seen. Physical examination may be unrevealing; however, in the presence of a severe contusion, inspiratory rales and decreased breath sounds may be found. A chest radiograph shows singular or multiple patchy alveolar infiltrates caused by intra-alveolar hemorrhage [6]. These patchy infiltrates can coalesce into homogenous infiltrates that involve a lobe or an entire lung. CT scans of the chest have been shown to be more sensitive in demonstrating the changes seen with pulmonary contusions than are routine chest radiographs [5]. In patients with pulmonary contusions, arterial PaO_2, alveolar arterial oxygen gradients, and pulmonary compliance are usually abnormally low. Hyperventilation may induce hypocapnia and respiratory alkalosis [7]. If the contusion is massive or if aspiration, infection, or ARDS develops, carbon dioxide may be retained and respiratory acidosis may ensue.

Treatment

Patients with pulmonary contusions should be hospitalized for careful monitoring because they can become critically ill rapidly. Oxygen should be administered as necessary to maintain arterial oxygen saturation greater than 90%. Patient-controlled analgesia, intravenous or epidural, should be used as necessary to control pain. Vigorous chest physiotherapy is important to keep the airway clear and help prevent the

development of atelectasis. If ventilation is inadequate, intubation and mechanical ventilation are indicated. If large volumes of fluid are necessary for resuscitation, a pulmonary artery catheter should be positioned so that pulmonary artery pressures and pulmonary capillary wedge pressures can be measured.

The use of steroids and antibiotics is controversial. Some authorities advocate the use of high doses of steroids for a short time, whereas others believe that the use of steroids is not indicated [8]. Prophylactic antibiotics are used in some institutions; in others, antibiotics are used only when evidence of infection is present.

Pulmonary contusions are not innocuous injuries. In one series, 11% of patients with severe isolated pulmonary contusions died, whereas the mortality rate was much higher (22%) in patients with associated injuries [9]. ARDS developed in 17% of patients with isolated pulmonary contusions and in 78% of patients with two or more simultaneous associated injuries in other series [10].

Pulmonary lacerations

Pulmonary parenchymal lacerations, although seen more commonly after penetrating chest trauma, are also seen after blunt trauma. Although blood vessels and tracheobronchial passages may be disrupted, pneumothorax is in many cases the major problem, and bleeding is of minor consequence. If the laceration involves the visceral pleura and the communication with the pleural space remains patent, hemothorax, pneumothorax, or hemopneumothorax results. If the visceral pleura is torn but quickly seals, blood, air, or both can accumulate within the parenchyma and result in the development of a hematoma, cyst, or a cyst containing blood.

As a result of high-speed motor vehicle crashes, extensive pulmonary lacerations, occasionally with volvulous or torsion of the lung, are being encountered with increasing frequency. Such lacerations often are centrally located, are associated with severe chest wall injuries and pulmonary contusion, and disrupt large vessels and major bronchi.

Pulmonary hematoma

Pulmonary lacerations resulting from blunt or penetrating injuries may fill with blood, forming a pulmonary hematoma. The reported incidence of hematomas developing in pulmonary contusions has ranged from 4% to 11% [5,11]. Because hematomas are recognized infrequently in clinical situations, the true incidence is likely to be less. Despite an unimpressive radiographic appearance, the injury represents a significant collection of intraparenchymal blood. It may not become visible radiographically for 24 to 72 hours after trauma resuscitation, during which time it increases insidiously. Pulmonary hematomas generally do not interfere with gas exchange, nor do they produce significant intrapulmonary shunting. Nevertheless, a pulmonary hematoma is a major risk factor for infection and lung abscess formation [12]. The use of CT scans permits more accurate evaluation of hematomas than conventional radiographs. On CT scans, hematomas have been found to shrink less than 0.5 cm in 3 weeks, whereas on conventional radiographs, they are reported to resolve within 2 to 4 weeks of injury [5]. In the absence of previous radiographs, serial films, or serial CT scans demonstrating the evolution of the hematoma, the exact nature of the nodule or lesion may be unclear, and the possibility of a neoplasm must be considered. If the nodule remains stable after 4 weeks, showing no evidence of resolution, fine-needle aspiration of the nodule or surgical excision should be performed to establish the nature of the lesion [13].

Management

In most cases, pulmonary lacerations heal promptly after chest tube insertion without any significant long-lasting ill effects. Peripheral lacerations encountered at operation can be oversewn (pneumonorrhaphy), stapled, or wedged out. Extensive lacerations may be centrally located and may disrupt major vessels and bronchi. Resultant massive bleeding, large air leaks, and, although rarely seen, bronchopulmonary venous fistulas resulting in systemic air embolization require immediate operation. Proceeding to a thoracotomy is determined by the urgency of this situation, location of the injury, and structures presumed to be involved. Lately, more trauma centers are using thoracoscopy as a diagnostic or therapeutic procedure for pulmonary lacerations [14,15]; however, if a thoracotomy is required, hilar compression with the fingers and then with a large vascular clamp, such as a Satinsky or curved DeBakey, is used to control bleeding and air leak and to stop systemic air embolization. When the hilum is controlled, if embolization

has occurred, air is aspirated from the left side of the heart, aorta, and coronary arteries. The vascular and bronchial injuries are then repaired, if possible, and the laceration is left open and drained with appropriately placed chest tubes.

Torsion or volvulous of the lobe or lung suggested by atypically oriented lobar collapse also necessitates prompt diagnosis and operation. At thoracotomy, the involved lobe or lung is untwisted and observed to ensure viability. If there is any question about its viability, the lobe or lung should be resected. Otherwise, the involved lobe should be stapled, if possible, to an adjacent lobe to prevent retwisting.

If a pulmonary hematoma or pulmonary contusion is identified at the time of thoracotomy, the surgeon should resist the temptation to resect the involved lung. Despite the gross appearance, there is rarely an indication for resection of an injured lung, unless there is associated significant injury to the airway or pulmonary vessels [16].

Pulmonary vascular injury

Vascular injury within the pulmonary parenchyma occurs within a low pressure system compressed by the surrounding parenchyma. Such hemorrhage generally stops with complete expansion of the lung [16,17]; however, uncorrected injury to the main pulmonary arteries or veins or to their principle lobar branches is usually lethal from rapid exsanguination because these structures bleed freely into the pleural space. Major pulmonary vascular injuries usually result from sudden deceleration. Mortalities rates for pulmonary arterial or venous injuries exceed 75%; therefore, the majority of these patients rarely survive long enough to reach a trauma center.

Management

If a major pulmonary vascular injury is diagnosed or suspected, control may be obtained at the pulmonary hilum by clamping the entire hilum. Through a thoracotomy incision, the hilum of the lung is grasped firmly with one hand as the surgeon uses the other hand to apply a long vascular clamp across the entire pulmonary hilum. This maneuver excludes the main pulmonary artery and veins from the circulation, may prevent exsanguination, and provides time for the anesthesiologist to resuscitate the patient. If there is a significant amount of blood in the airway, a double-lumen endotracheal tube or a bronchial blocker may be used to protect the opposite lung from aspiration of blood. Next, the vascular injury should be isolated and repaired using standard vascular techniques [18]. If a lobar pulmonary artery is irreparable, it may be ligated without fear of pulmonary necrosis. The bronchial blood supply is usually sufficient to maintain parenchymal viability. If the venous drainage to a parenchymal region must be sacrificed, the involved parenchyma should be resected to prevent infarction of that portion of the lung secondary to venous obstruction [18].

Video-assisted thoracic surgery or thoracoscopy

Although most chest traumas do not require a major operation, tube thoracostomy remains the basis of treatment. Patients who would have required a thoracotomy in the past may actually benefit from a less invasive surgical technique to perform diagnostic and therapeutic procedures after blunt chest trauma. Improvements in instrumentation, especially endoscopic staplers and cameras, and endoscopic surgical techniques have expanded the indications for video-assisted thoracic surgery (VATS) or thoracoscopy in the diagnosis and treatment of diseases within the chest; however, the use of VATS remains controversial in trauma patients. Early publications explored the use of VATS in patients sustaining thoracic trauma [19,20]. The results were encouraging, but the series reported a small number of cases. In 1999, a meta-analysis of the use of thoracoscopy in trauma was published that involved 28 studies and more than 500 patients. The complication rate was 2% and the missed injury rate 0.8%. The most important benefit was that 62% of patients did not require a thoracotomy or laparotomy for diagnosis or treatment of their thoracic injuries [21]. VATS is an accurate and effective modality in the evaluation and management of hemodynamically stable patients who experience thoracic injuries. One should have a low threshold to perform an open procedure if the situation arises. A relative stable thoracic trauma patient can become extremely unstable at any moment; therefore, one should be prepared to proceed with a thoracotomy immediately. Caution should also be taken in the thoracic trauma patient with multiple injuries, especially severe intra-abdominal injuries.

Blunt thoracic trauma continues to be a significant cause of morbidity and mortality in the United States. A comprehensive evaluation of these patients is needed to improve their survival. Understanding the lung injuries that can occur related to blunt chest trauma is essential to improved outcomes. The use of VATS in blunt thoracic trauma has improved the diagnosis and management of patients with life-threatening pulmonary injuries.

References

[1] Breasted JH. The Edwin Smith surgical papyrus, vol. 1. Chicago: University of Chicago Press; 1930.
[2] Withington ET [translator]. Hippocrates, vol. 3. Cambridge (MA): Harvard University Press; 1959. [99, 307–13].
[3] Wiot J. The radiographic manifestations of blunt chest trauma. JAMA 1975;231:500–3.
[4] Chopra P, Kroncke G, Berkoff H, et al. Pulmonary contusion: a problem in blunt chest trauma. Wis Med J 1977;76:S1–3.
[5] Wagner RB, Crawford WO Jr, Schimpf PP. Classification of parenchymal injuries of the lung. Radiology 1998;167:77–82.
[6] Stevens E, Templeton A. Traumatic nonpenetrating lung contusions. Radiology 1965;85:247–52.
[7] Erikson D, Shinozaki T, Beekman E, et al. Relationship of arterial blood gases and pulmonary radiographs to the degree of pulmonary contusion. J Trauma 1971;11:689–94.
[8] Svennevig J, Bugge-Asperheim B, Birkeland S, et al. Efficacy of steroids in the treatment of lung contusion. Acta Chir Scand Suppl 1980;499:87–92.
[9] Demuth WE Jr, Smith JM. Pulmonary contusion. Am Surg 1965;109:819–23.
[10] Pepe P, Potkin R, Reus D, et al. Clinical predictors of the adult respiratory distress syndrome. Am J Surg 1982;144:124–30.
[11] Westermark N. A roentgenological investigation into traumatic lung changes arisen through blast violence to the thorax. Acta Radiol 1941;22:331.
[12] Hankins J, Attar S, Turndy S, et al. Differential diagnosis of pulmonary parenchymal changes in thoracic trauma. Am Surg 1973;39:309–18.
[13] Engelman RM, Boyd AD, Blum M, et al. Multiple circumscribed pulmonary hematomas masquerading as metastatic carcinoma. Ann Thorac Surg 1973;15:291–4.
[14] Abolhoda A, Livingston DH, Donahoo JS, et al. Diagnostic and therapeutic video assisted thoracic surgery (VATS) following chest trauma. Eur J Cardiothorac Surg 1997;12:356–60.
[15] Manlulu AV, Lee TW, Thung KH, et al. Current indications and results of VATS in the evaluation and management of hemodynamically stable thoracic injuries. Eur J Cardiothorac Surg 2004;25:1048–53.
[16] Graham JM, Mattox KL, Beall AC. Penetrating trauma of the lung. J Trauma 1979;19:655–9.

[17] Beall AC, Crawford HW, Debakey ME. Considerations in the management of acute traumatic hemothorax. J Thorac Cardiovasc Surg 1966;52: 351–60.

[18] Carr RE. Injuries to the pulmonary parenchyma and vasculature. In: Daughtry DC, editor. Thoracic trauma. Boston: Little Brown; 1980.

[19] Smith RS, Fry WR, Tsoi EKM, et al. Preliminary report on videothoracoscopy in the evaluation and treatment of thoracic injury. Am J Surg 1993;166: 690–5.

[20] Kern JA, Tribble CG, Spotnitz WD, et al. Thoracoscopy in the subacute management of patients with thoracoabdominal trauma. Chest 1993;104: 942–5.

[21] Villavicencio RT, Aucar JA, Wall MR Jr. Analysis of thoracoscopy in trauma. Surg Endosc 1999; 13:3–9.

ELSEVIER
SAUNDERS

Thorac Surg Clin 17 (2007) 63–72

THORACIC
SURGERY
CLINICS

Esophageal Trauma

Ayesha S. Bryant, MSPH, MD[a], Robert J. Cerfolio, MD[b],*

[a]Department of Epidemiology, University of Alabama at Birmingham, 1900 University Boulevard,
712 Tinsley Harrison Tower, Birmingham, AL 65294, USA
[b]Department of Surgery, Division of Cardiothoracic Surgery, University of Alabama at Birmingham,
703 19th St. S, 2RB T39, Birmingham, AL 35294, USA

The incidence of blunt and penetrating trauma that leads to a proved esophagus injury is rare. This low incidence is probably related to several factors. First, most of this muscular tubular-organ that connects the laryngopharynx to the stomach is housed in the well-protected posterior mediastinum. The hard bony shell of the thoracic cavity and the position of the esophagus deep within it prevent many injuries. Second, the diagnosis of small or contained perforations may go undiagnosed secondary to other more serious vascular injuries that require urgent attention. Third, many esophageal traumas may be associated with lethal vascular injuries in patients who never survive the trip to the emergency room. The upper most proximal third of the esophagus, the cervical portion, however, lies in the neck and is susceptible to sharp or penetrating trauma. The grading of esophageal injuries is shown in Table 1.

The treatment of blunt or sharp traumatic injuries to the esophageal depends on several factors: the timing of the injury; the degree of injury (contained perforation compared with non-contained perforation); and the location of the injury. Because the location is a critical factor in the treatment and the selected surgical approach, a brief review of esophageal anatomy is necessary for adequate therapy and is provided first. The remainder of this article provides information on the methods of injury, the diagnosis, and different treatment strategies for traumatic esophageal injuries. In addition, because other types of esophageal trauma are more commonly seen and treated than those from blunt or penetrating

trauma, also provided is a brief synopsis of iatrogenic and corrosive esophageal injures. The principles applied in the management of these types of injuries can and should be applied to all types of esophageal insults.

Anatomy

The esophagus lies posterior to the trachea and the heart and passes through the posterior mediastinum by the esophageal hiatus. It traverses through this diaphragmatic opening at the level of the T10 vertebral body on its decent from the thoracic cavity into the abdomen. The esophagus is not just a passive muscular tube. It is a functional, highly innervated, dynamic organ that actively propels particulate matter and liquid from the mouth to the stomach. Unlike most of the digestive tract, it has no mesentery and no serosal coating; tissue around the esophagus is called the adventitia. There are no large neurovascular or fibrous structures that tether the esophagus within the chest. This lends the esophagus amenable to blunt stripping from the mediastinum. This lack of tethering probably helps prevent the esophagus from tearing or disruption during sudden deceleration injuries, like those that occur in the aorta and the carina or main stem bronchi tree.

The esophagus is the narrowest part of the gastrointestinal tract. It originates at the distal end of the laryngopharynx, at the level of the sixth cervical vertebra. It terminates by widening to form the stomach, the most voluminous part of the gastrointestinal tract. The esophagus is flat in its upper and middle parts and rounded in its lower part. When distended, these parts present

* Corresponding author.
E-mail address: rcerfolio@uab.edu (R.J. Cerfolio).

Table 1
Types of penetrating injuries by location

Cervical esophagus
Iatrogenic (endoscopy, dilatation)
Endotracheal intubation
Gunshot wound
Ingestion of a foreign body
Perforation of Zenker's diverticulum
Stab wounds
Lye ingestion
Upper thoracic
Iatrogenic (endoscopy dilatation, biopsy)
Gunshot wound
Lye ingestion
Lower thoracic esophagus
Iatrogenic (endoscopy, biopsy, dilatation)
Ingestion of foreign body
Vagotomy
Spontaneous (postemetic)
Abdominal esophagus
Iatrogenic (paraesophageal surgery)
Spontaneous (postemetic)

diameters of only 2.5 × 1.6 cm and 2.5 × 2.4 cm, respectively. The esophageal tube collapses when at rest and ranges in size from 0.6 to 1.5 cm in diameter. This relatively small size makes it less likely to be struck with a high-speed missile. The average length of the esophagus between the cricoid cartilage and cardiac notch of the gastro-esophageal junction ranges from 21 to 34 cm (27 cm average). The cervical portion of the esophagus is about 3 to 5 cm in length, the thoracic esophagus is 18 to 22 cm long, and the abdominal part is about 3 to 6 cm in length (Fig. 1). In practice, clinicians usually measure abnormalities within the esophagus by stating its distance from the incisors. This anatomic landmark is also used for manometric and endoscopic procedures. The most commonly used distances are the cricoid cartilage, which is 13 to 16 cm from the incisors; the carina, which is 23 to 26 cm from the incisors; and the gastroesophageal junction, which is 39 to 48 cm from the incisors [1,2].

Penetrating trauma

Penetrating injuries are secondary to many types of objects, but can be separated into four main types of injuries. The first is from a sharp weapon, such as a knife, and the second is from a high-speed projectile, such as a bullet. These types of penetrating injuries are less commonly seen than the third and the fourth types. The third type of traumatic penetrating injury is an iatrogenic laceration or trauma from a scope or from esophageal dilation. The fourth type of penetrating trauma comes from the lumen outward, as opposed to the other three types, which come from muscular coat inward. This last type of penetrating trauma is a laceration to the mucosal surface of the esophagus, such as from the ingestion of a sharp foreign object like a razor or pit. Lye ingestion represents an example of this type of injury because it injures the mucosal surface first and can lead to full-thickness necrosis with or without perforation later. The incidence and characteristics of these four types of penetrating traumas are described next. Table 1 summarizes the different mechanisms of penetrating esophageal injuries by anatomic locations.

Impaling objects (knife wound)

The most common part of the esophagus that is injured from an impaling weapon-like injury is the cervical esophagus [3–5]. Like any patients who presents with a stab injury, injuries to other surrounding structures also must be investigated and ruled out. In the neck this includes the pharynx, larynx, trachea, and the carotid arteries and jugular veins. The clinical status of the patient dictates the treatment algorithm. In a patient who is clinically stable and has no hemodynamic instability, the esophagus is best evaluated with a radiologic swallow study using Gastrografin. A negative Gastrografin swallow test does not eliminate an esophageal injury, because false-negative tests have been reported in up to 10% of perforations [6,7]. A negative test usually provides evidence that surgical intervention is not indicated, however, at least not initially.

High-speed missile (gunshot wound)

As the lethality of weapons on the streets and in the battlefield has increased, the incidence of esophageal injuries from gunshot wounds has also increased. Many patients, however, succumb to concomitant vascular injures before any required intervention for their esophageal injury. Interestingly, late perforation secondary to full-thickness necrosis from these types of weapons may also be more likely.

Iatrogenic injury, endoscopic perforation

Perforation of the esophagus can be caused by the passage of any instrument or object (Table 2)

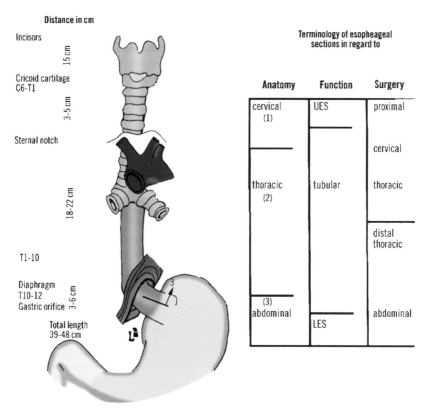

Fig. 1. Anatomy of the esophagus relative to clinically important structures.

[8]. The major causes of instrumental perforation are diagnostic endoscopic procedures and the dilatation of esophageal strictures. The common sites for instrumental perforations are the pyriform fossa, the part of the esophagus that crosses under the aortic arch, the lower third just proximal to the esophagogastric junction, or a region of a stricture or pathology. The extent of the perforation governs the therapy and the timing of the

diagnosis and the clinical status of the patient. There are several degrees of perforation: acute intrapleural perforation, which almost always requires immediate surgical intervention; subacute mediastinal and delayed intrapleural rupture, which can often be managed with percutaneous drainage and observation; intramural perforation, which can be managed with observation; and intra-abdominal perforations, which almost always require urgent surgical intervention.

Foreign body and mucosal injures (lye ingestion)

Mucosal injury to the esophagus can be a result of the ingestion of foreign bodies or caustic agents. The severity and extent of esophageal and gastric damage resulting from a caustic ingestion depends on several factors. These factors include the corrosive properties of the ingested substance; the amount ingested; the concentration of the ingested material; the physical form (solid or liquid) of the agent; and the duration of contact with the mucosa. Suicidal patients often ingest larger amounts of caustic agents than those who

Table 2
Incidence of esophageal perforation by procedure type

Esophageal dilation	0.5%
Esophageal dilation for achalasia	1.7%
Endoscopic thermal therapy	1%–2%
Endoscopic variceal sclerotherapy	1%–6%
Endoscopic laser therapy	5%
Esophageal photodynamic therapy	4.6%
Esophageal stent placement	5%–25%

From Infatolino A, Ter RB. Rupture and perforation of the esophagus. In: Castell DO, Richter JE, editors. The esophagus. 3rd edition. Philadelphia: Lippincott Williams & Wilkins; 1999. p. 597; with permission.

accidentally swallow these agents; as a result, they are likely to have more severe esophageal and gastric damage. These injuries need to be carefully identified and early endoscopy can document the extent of the damage and the severity of the damage.

Swallowing injuries to the esophagus can be produced by a wide array of foreign objects including batteries, food bolus, pills, and pins. Fig. 2 displays a contained perforation from a glass shard. Bone fragments are the most commonly swallowed foreign bodies in adults that lead to esophageal trauma. Trauma may be induced by laceration or by perforation during attempted passage. Incarcerated foreign body in a healthy esophagus is usually located in the cervical esophagus. When incarceration occurs in the lower esophagus, an esophageal disease should be suspected. Removal using endoscopic techniques is best and the underlying pathology should also be treated.

Signs and symptoms of perforation

The typical clinical presentation of traumatic esophageal perforation is acute dysphagia or the inability to swallow saliva [9]. The most common clinical features in a review of 103 patients with a history of foreign body ingestion were dysphagia (92%) and tenderness in neck (60%) [10]. Inability to swallow oral secretions is an important symptom because it indicates total esophageal obstruction. Other symptoms that can occur include hypersalivation, retrosternal fullness, regurgitation of undigested food, and occasionally odynophagia. Most adults with incarceration of a foreign body present with a painful sensation around the lower jugular notch that is aggravated by swallowing. The pain does not necessarily reflect the position of the foreign body or damage; pain is often felt higher than the actual sight of incarceration.

Diagnosis and treatment

A lateral radiograph of the cervical and upper thoracic regions should be ordered to look for the foreign body and also to check for any mediastinal emphysema secondary to a perforation. Despite a normal soft tissue radiograph and the lack of mediastinal emphysema, if a high degree of suspicion persists, an upper gastrointestinal swallow should be ordered using Gastrografin. Some recommend esophagoscopy, but the authors favor this only after a swallow that provides anatomic information has been performed. Endoscopy can be performed for visualization and attempted extraction. A relative contraindication against esophagoscopy is presence of severe hematemesis, which indicates possible vascular lesion caused by a deeply impacted and perforating foreign body [11].

Ingestion of caustic substances is usually accidental in children under the age of 5 years and intentional in adults and adolescents. The most caustic ingestion is the swallowing of a strong alkali (sodium or potassium hydroxide) contained in drain cleaners, other household cleaning products, or disc batteries. The term "lye" implies substances that contain sodium or potassium

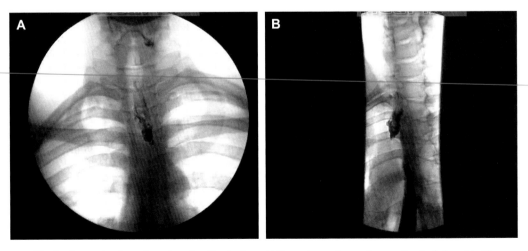

Fig. 2. A contained esophageal perforation in the mid thoracic esophagus from a shard of glass (*A*, *B*).

hydroxide. Highly concentrated acids (hydrochloric, sulfuric, and phosphoric) contained in toilet bowl or swimming pool cleaners, antirust compounds, or in battery fluid are less frequently ingested. Button batteries contain highly concentrated alkaline solutions. Damage can occur from the release of the alkali, local electrical current discharge, and direct pressure necrosis from the foreign body. When lodged in the esophagus, burns can occur within 4 hours and perforation within 6 hours; urgent endoscopy is indicated in this setting.

Blunt trauma

Blunt trauma to the esophagus refers to an injury secondary to a force that is not contiguous with the esophagus but injuries it indirectly. This includes barotrauma, which is defined by rapid changes in the pressure in the esophageal lumen that leads to perforation or laceration of the esophageal wall. These injuries are probably more common than thought and often go unrecognized, often because patients succumb to other more lethal types of injuries sustained at the same time. Table 3 summarizes some of the common causes of blunt esophageal injuries. Several examples of each type are also provided.

Blunt injuries

Blunt trauma to the esophagus may be caused by a forceful or crushing esophageal injury, such as those associated with motor vehicle accidents or when a patient is struck in the neck by the steering wheel. It also includes blows to the head during a boxing match and even esophageal injuries sustained during the Heimlich maneuver or cardiopulmonary resuscitation.

In blunt trauma, direct esophageal injury most often occurs at the thoracic outlet. It can result from a deceleration injury that tears the esophagus against the vertebral bodies or from fracture dislocation of the vertebrae. A common mechanism is the steering wheel injury, in which the sternum is driven back against the thoracic spine. In older subjects, this is often associated with

Table 3
Common causes of blunt esophageal trauma

Barotrauma
Mallory-Weiss tear
Gunshot
Crush injury (motor vehicle accident)

multiple bilateral rib fractures. The posterior wall of the trachea may be split longitudinally, resulting in extensive mediastinal emphysema and pneumothoraces. The tracheal injury may accompany extensive trauma to the upper third of the intrathoracic esophagus, consisting of extensive vertical lacerations. The esophageal injury is frequently obscured by the chest wall, and airway injury and may not be recognized until a swallow is ordered. A high index of suspicious is necessary and should accompany any type of blunt injury that leads to a major airway injury. An esophageal injury should also be suspected when swallowing provokes violent coughing and chest roentgenogram shows rapidly increasing bilateral pleural effusions.

Tracheoesophageal fistula can develop over time from blunt trauma. The finding of air in the mediastinum is not unusual in the patient who has sustained significant blunt trauma, but it is not specific for esophageal or tracheal injury. Contrast studies are needed, as is bronchoscopy to evaluate each system.

Barotrauma

Barotrauma of the esophagus is caused by rapid transmural changes in pressure in the lumen of the esophagus. Types of injuries that may cause barotrauma include blast injuries, accidental misdirection of a compressed air nozzle, aggressive attempts to resuscitate neonates by face mask using a high-pressure oxygen source, and Boerhaave's syndrome. During Boerhaave's, the patient vomits against a closed glottis, which results in an increase in intraluminal esophageal pressure, ultimately leading to a perforation. Barotrauma from blast injuries are increasingly occurring and have been seen with soldiers in the war in Iraq.

Other similar type of barotrauma injuries include Mallory-Weiss tear, which is usually caused by vomiting, retching, or vigorous coughing. The tear usually involves the gastric mucosa near the squamocolumnar mucosal junction. Patients present with upper gastrointestinal bleeding, which may be severe, and commonly there develops a left pleural effusion. In most patients bleeding ceases spontaneously; continued bleeding may respond to vasopressin therapy or angiographic embolization.

Diagnosis

A complete history and physical examination is an integral part of making the diagnosis of an esophageal injury. A high index of suspicion is important. The history from the patient or from an observer, if the patient is noncommunicative, should be elicited to determine the mechanism of injury. The physical examination can yield important clues that suggest an esophageal injury, such as subcutaneous emphysema. Other findings include tachypnea, tachycardia, and fever, which are associated with extravasation of the esophageal contents into the mediastinum.

Laboratory studies

Perforating injuries can cause abnormal results of several laboratory tests attributed to an inflammatory response, including a rapid increase in the leukocyte count and left shift; low PO_2; and acidosis on arterial blood gas results (as a result of reaction of extravasation of esophageal contents or impairment of respiratory function by extravasation into one or both pleural spaces). Lactic acid can also be elevated. Serum electrolytes may be elevated because of hemoconcentration caused by fluid loss secondary to the inflammatory response. Analysis of a pleural effusion that is formed by an esophageal perforation is not only consistent with an exudate, but may also show hyperamylesemia.

Sagittal cervical films show streaks of air in the soft tissue planes; chest radiographs may show pneumomediastinum and posterior-superior mediastinal pleural fluid collections. Often, right-sided pleural effusion develops in patients who do not receive surgical treatment within 24 hours once the perforation leaks into the right pleural space.

Swallow studies

The mainstay for establishing the diagnosis of an esophageal injury is by contrast swallow studies. Gastrografin should be used first, and then if there is no evidence of a leak, barium can be used. There is much information that can be gleaned from an esophageal swallow study, such as the specifics of the peristaltic waves of the esophagus, the presence or absence of extrinsic compression, dilation of the esophagus, and so forth. In a true trauma setting, however, only the presence or absence of a leak is the information that is truly needed. One must remember that there is a false-negative rate for Gastrografin swallows, and even those followed by barium. A negative test does not definitively mean there is no leak; however, it supports an initial nonoperative

approach unless there are other signs or symptoms that suggest the test is false-negative. Then, a repeat study should be performed.

The Gastrografin swallow test is positive in about 60% to 80% of patients with a cervical perforation [12]. Figs. 3–8 illustrate the different types and locations of perforations. A thin barium swallow or esophagoscopy may demonstrate the perforation in patients who are symptomatic yet have a negative Gastrografin swallow study. Esophagoscopy is indicated in cases of foreign body perforation or penetrating trauma. Some recommend esophagoscopy further to diagnosis a leak. This carries the risk of making the leak larger, however, or converting a contained leak into a noncontained leak. Air is insufflated into the esophagus during flexible esophagoscopy and rigid scope, which do not require air to be carefully performed. Series have shown that esophagoscopy has a sensitivity of 100% and specificity of 83% in locating the injury [12,13]. The authors prefer radiologic test over esophagoscopy.

Treatment: overview

Treatment of a traumatic esophageal injury is dictated by many factors, which include the patient's hemodynamic stability, associated injuries, other planned operative interventions, and so forth. The remainder of this section considers a patient who is hemodynamically stable, has no other injuries, has no contraindications to urgent

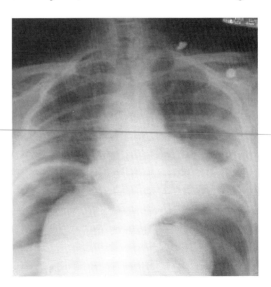

Fig. 3. Free air under diaphragm secondary to an abdominal esophageal perforation after dilatation.

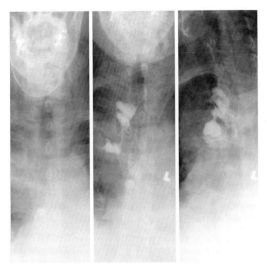

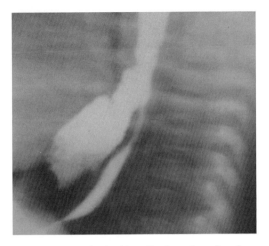

Fig. 6. Noncontained mid to distal esophageal perforation following attempted dilatation (iatrogenic).

Fig. 4. Noncontained upper to mid thoracic esophageal perforation into the right mediastinum.

surgery, and who is able to tolerate and undergo all types of surgical approaches.

The decision to operate or whether to observe a patient who is stable with an esophageal injury is multifactorial. The degree or extent of the esophageal injury is critical in the decision making. If the swallow study shows a noncontained perforation, defined as the extravasation of

Gastrografin or other contrast material or dye into the pleural space, surgical intervention is required. The goals of the operation in this situation are removal of all infected fluid and material; decortication of the lung; identification of the perforation (if possible); and primary repair and buttressing with autologous tissue. Tissue that can be used includes a pedicled intercostal muscle flap, a pedicled pericardial flap, a pedicled diaphragmatic patch, pericardial fat, or pleural.

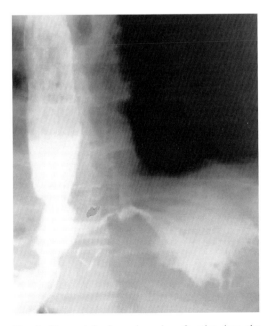

Fig. 5. Noncontained esophageal perforation into the left pleural space.

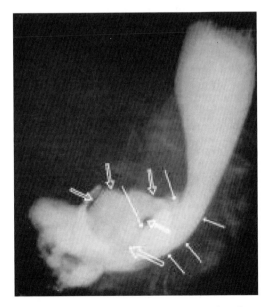

Fig. 7. A contained distal thoracic esophageal perforation after dilation of a benign reflux-induced stricture. Arrows indicate sites of contained perforation.

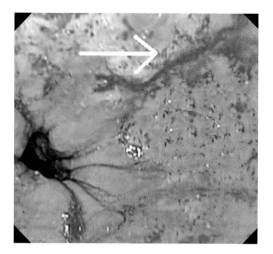

Fig. 8. Endoscopic view of a Boerhaave's tear (*arrow*).

The latter is often too thin and is not an ideal choice.

If there has been a greater than 24-hour time delay between the injury and the radiologic diagnosis, the infected effusion stills need to be completely drained, but urgent exploration may not be needed in properly selected patients. There are several methods that can be used to achieve drainage of the pleural space: a chest tube, a video-assisted thoracoscopic procedure, or even percutaneous drainage. The authors prefer a video-assisted thoracoscopic procedure to ensure the entire effusion is drained, all particulate material is removed, the lung is decorticated, and the chest is thoroughly washed out with many liters of warm saline or water so chest tubes can be perfectly positioned. These basic principals should be followed. The concept of surgical repair based on the location of the leak is reviewed later.

Cervical esophageal leak

Most patients with cervical esophageal perforations complain of neck pain that is worsened by neck flexion and dysphagia and odynophagia. There may be tenderness and crepitus in the neck on palpation. Fever and leukocytosis develop promptly. Over two thirds of cervical esophageal perforations are caused by endoscopy; the remainder is caused by penetrating trauma. Cervical esophageal leaks that are diagnosed near the time of the injury should be treated with exploration, usually through a neck incision or collar incision.As soon as a cervical esophageal perforation is suspected, the patient should receive nothing by mouth, a nasogastric tube placed, and

treatment with intravenous antibiotics started. Commonly used antibiotics are those that provide empiric coverage for anaerobic and both gram-negative and gram-positive aerobes. Clindamycin remains a mainstay of therapy. Once the patient is stabilized and associated injuries are eliminated, surgical treatment in the form of cervical drainage should be initiated promptly. The authors prefer a left neck incision parallel to the left sternocleidomastoid muscle. The principles of the operation are the same: debridement of all infected tissue, closure of the defect primarily with local muscle patching, and drainage of the wound. Leaks in the neck can be managed by drainage only. Identification of the leak is not always necessary as long as the infected material is removed, drains are placed, and viable tissue and neck muscles are left intact abutting the cervical esophagus to help seal the unidentified leak.

Thoracic esophageal leak

Thoracic perforations occur most commonly from iatrogenic injuries. Other causes include barotrauma, caustic ingestion, cancer, and penetrating wounds. Iatrogenic perforations are often a result of insufficient sedation, repeated attempts to dilate strictures, attempted dilation of stricture for achalasia, and biopsies performed under poor visualization.

Noncontained perforation after dilation of esophageal stricture

A noncontained perforation in a patient with a stricture is a special circumstance that requires careful thought before embarking on surgery. If biopsies were taken before the dilation that caused the perforation, the surgeon should wait for the result of the biopsies. The pathologist should be called and asked to interpret the tissue as quickly as possible. Often one can wait 6 to 12 hours safely without harming the patient, but each clinical situation needs to be carefully assessed. If waiting is unwise, or if biopsies were not taken and the index of suspicion for a malignant stricture is high, the operative approach should start in the chest. The chest that contains the pleural effusion should be opened by thoracotomy. The operative principals described previously should be followed but in addition, biopsies of the stricture should be performed and frozen sections sent to pathology. If the operation occurs at night or early in the morning, the pathologist should be called before the surgery and as the operative team is assembled so he or she is aware that they are needed. This strategy prevents a malignant stricture from being repaired instead of resected, and unnecessary delays during the operation. If the diagnosis of cancer is known before surgery, the operation can start in the abdomen and then finish in the chest. If the diagnosis is not known, the operation should start in the affected chest and biopsies of the stricture performed. If the stricture is benign, a stricturoplasty should be performed and the perforation repaired and then buttressed. If the biopsies are malignant, the esophagus should be resected. The esophagus should be freed, lymph nodes removed, the empyema drained, the lung decorticated, the chest closed, and the operation finished with the patient supine. A transhiatal esophagogastrectomy is than performed and a feeding jejunostomy inserted.

Signs, symptoms, and diagnosis

Perforation of the thoracic esophagus is clinically manifested by substernal or epigastric pain, mediastinal emphysema, and pleural effusion. Most patients with a thoracic perforation do not present with subcutaneous air. A Gastrografin swallow should be performed.

Boerhaave (see Fig. 3) first described postemetic esophageal perforation in 1704, and today the term is used to describe emesis-induced esophageal perforation. It is typically seen in alcoholics but can occur in any patient with severe vomiting or retching. It is caused by an acute pressure rise in the esophagus from forceful vomiting against a closed glottis. Rupture typically occurs at the left aspect of the gastroesophageal junction with extravasation of gastric contents into the mediastinum and into the lower left pleural space. The diagnosis should be suspected in anyone with severe chest pain and dyspnea following forceful vomiting, especially if they have a left pleural effusion. Associated findings may include cervical crepitus caused by pneumomediastinum and sepsis induced by the subsequent mediastinitis.

If the diagnosis of a noncontained traumatic esophageal perforation is made soon after the injury has occurred (within 12 hours), immediate exploration by thoracotomy is best. The side the contrast material drains into is the best side to open. The goals of the operation are to evacuate all infected material; decorticate the lung so it can completely expand; locate the esophageal tear; debride all devitalized tissue; and patch the defect with viable tissue (intercostal muscle harvested before rib spreading, diaphragmatic muscle, pericardial fat, pericardial patch, and so forth). The

defect should be closed primarily if after debridement its lumen is not compromised. A dilator should be placed and closure performed over it if needed to ensure an adequate lumen. The autologous pedicled flap should be placed as a supplement over the primary repair.

Abdominal esophageal leak

Perforation of the abdominal esophagus is rare because of its short segment. Iatrogenic injuries and spontaneous ruptures that lead into the chest are most common. If suspected, the diagnosis should be confirmed by a Gastrografin swallow. More commonly, the diagnosis is made by the presence of free-air on an abdominal flat-plate or by CT. A free perforation into the peritoneal cavity requires operative intervention. The principals of the operation include an upper midline incision; irrigation of the entire peritoneal cavity, especially of the subphrenic areas on both sides; and repair of the injury. The stomach can be used to buttress the repair, but it should not be circumferentially wrapped around the esophagus because manometric studies have rarely been performed before this urgent operation. A feeding jejunostomy tube should also be placed at the time of repair and other abdominal injuries should be sought for and treated. If the patient has malignancy, a careful exploration of the abdomen (the liver, omentum, and so forth) should be inspected to rule out metastatic lesions, and lymph nodes also should be removed.

Diversion

In rare situations, exploration may reveal a necrotic esophagus. This is almost always seen in patients who have prolonged time intervals (36 hours or greater) between injury and exploration and in those who suffered severe trauma. This situation is exceedingly rare. The authors have never encountered this situation, yet have seen many patients who have had diversion performed. Before deciding that resection with diversion is needed, the surgeon should ensure the complete lack of viability of the esophageal tissue because this is so rarely seen. Many surgeons too quickly choose this option and perform unnecessary diversions and create a difficult problem later for those patients who survive. This option does not lead to increased survival and merely obviates the need for repair, which too many surgeons are unwilling to attempt. Cervical esophagostomy is too frequently performed. Moreover, the placement of multiple tubes, such as T tubes or drains or fabricated concoctions in the defunctionalized remaining esophagus, unnecessarily complicates reconstruction later. There are not needed.

Most heavily infected chest can be debrided and the entire esophagus salvaged. The continuity of the esophagus should be preserved in 99% of patients. In the very rare situation that this is not possible and diversion has to be performed, all necrotic material should be resected. The remaining length of the stomach and esophagus should be maximized. The end of the diverted esophagus should be drained by an end esophagostomy (there is little role for a partially diverting side esophagostomy). It should be placed as far inferiorly (below the clavicle) as possible. The esophagus should be tunneled subcutaneously anterior to the clavicle but positioned inferiorly to it so a stomal-appliance bag can be placed on it more easily. This bag is more easily hidden and works better on the chest than on the neck. The remaining esophagus should be left in place in the posterior mediastinum so that route can be used 6 to 12 months later when definitive reconstruction using the stomach or colon is performed. The distal end of the esophagus should be stapled and the mucous secretion allowed to drain distally into the stomach. Tubes do not need to be placed in this limb; however, they are often unnecessarily placed. The authors frequently encounter tubes in this limb. Once the chest is treated and closed the patient should be placed supine, reprepared and draped, and a midline upper abdominal incision made. A gastrostomy tube should be placed along with a feeding jejunostomy tube. After the patient is fully recovered and has undergone rehabilitation, which usually takes at least 6 months, gastrointestinal continuity can be re-established using a gastric or colon interposition graft.

Summary

Injury from blunt or penetrating trauma to the esophagus is relatively rare. Treatment strategy is contingent on the clinical status of the patient, associated injuries, and the degree of esophageal injury and the time of injury until diagnosis. Although nonoperative intervention may be acceptable in highly selected patients with contained injuries or those who are more than 24 hours removed from the injury and are clinically stable, operative intervention is the most conservative and safest approach. There are many potential surgical approaches but resection or diversion should be discouraged. Operative approaches include either side of the neck or chest, and an abdominal approach for selected injuries. Sometimes combined incisions are needed. The goal of any operation for a traumatic esophageal injury is removal of infected material, debridement of the esophagus, assessment of the distal and proximal extent of the injury, decortication of the lung if the injury soils the pleural space, primary closure of the esophageal defect if possible with buttressing of the closure with autologous pedicles tissue or muscle flaps, and to ensure distal patency without esophageal pathology.

References

[1] Liebermann-Meffert D, Duranceau A. Anatomy and embryology. In: Orringer MB, Zuidema GD, editors. Shackelford's surgery of the alimentary tract (4th edition). The esophagus, vol. I. Philadelphia: WB Saunders; 1996. p. 3–38.
[2] Liebermann-Meffert D. Anatomy, embryology, and histology. In: Pearson FG, Deslauriers J, Ginsberg RJ, editors. Esophageal surgery. New York: Churchill Livingstone; 1996. p. 1–25.
[3] Cohn HE, Hubbard A, Patton G. Management of esophageal injuries. Ann Thorac Surg 1989;48: 309–14.
[4] Wood J, Fabian TC, Mangiante EC. Penetrating neck injuries: recommendations for selecting management. J Trauma 1989;29:602–9.
[5] Yap RG, Yap AG, Obeid FN, et al. Traumatic esophageal injuries: 12-year experience at Henry Ford Hospital. J Trauma 1984;24:623–5.
[6] Sarr MG, Pemberton JH, Payne WS. Management of instrumental perforations of the esophagus. J Thorac Cardiovasc Surg 1982;84:211–8.
[7] Phillips LG Jr, Cunningham J. Esophageal perforation. Radiol Clin North Am 1984;22:607–13.
[8] Infatolino A, Ter RB. Rupture and perforation of the esophagus. In: Castell DO, Richter JE, editors. The esophagus. 3rd edition. Philadelphia: Lippincott Williams & Wilkins; 1999. p. 595–605.
[9] Nandi P, Ong GB. Foreign body in the oesophagus: review of 2394 cases. Br J Surg 1978;65:5–9.
[10] Khan MA, Hameed A, Choudhry AJ. Management of foreign bodies in the esophagus. J Coll Physicians Surg Pak 2004;14:218–20.
[11] Besson A, Meyer A, Savary M, et al. Study of 58 intrathoracic complications in 166 accidental or iatrogenic esophageal injuries. Schweiz Med Wochenschr 1981;111(43):1602–7.
[12] Armstrong WB, Detar TR, Stanley RB. Diagnosis and management of external penetrating esophageal injuries. Ann Otol Rhinol Laryngol 1994;103: 868–71.
[13] Horwitz B, Krevosky B, Buckman RF, et al. Endoscopic evaluation of penetrating esophageal injuries. Am J Gastroenterol 1993;88:1249–53.

ELSEVIER
SAUNDERS

Thorac Surg Clin 17 (2007) 73–79

THORACIC
SURGERY
CLINICS

Video-Assisted Thoracic Surgical Applications in Thoracic Trauma

Ibrahim B. Cetindag, MD[a], Todd Neideen, MD[b],
Stephen R. Hazelrigg, MD[a],*

[a]Department of Surgery, Southern Illinois University School of Medicine, 800 North Rutledge,
Room D319, Springfield, IL 62794-9638, USA
[b]Department of Surgery, Medical College of Wisconsin, 8701 Watertown Plank Road,
Milwaukee, WI 53226, USA

Thoracic trauma accounts for approximately 25% of trauma-related deaths [1–3]. A small number of patients with thoracic trauma either require emergency thoracotomy for life-threatening penetrating injury or urgent thoracotomy for aortic, esophageal, or tracheobronchial injury. The remaining 85% to 90% of thoracic trauma victims who reach the emergency room are treated with pain control, chest tube drainage, or pulmonary toilet [4,5]. Some of these patients may progress to develop acute and chronic complications that require operative therapy. For example, 18% to 30% of patients with a traumatic hemothorax have a retained hemothorax [5,6]. A traumatic pneumothorax may have a persistent airleak in 4% to 24% of patients [5,7]. Empyema may develop secondary to a retained hemothorax, persistent pneumothorax, missed diaphragm injury, or as a complication of hospital-acquired pneumonias. Delayed operative intervention may also be indicated for suspected diaphragmatic injuries.

Up until the late 1980s, many had pushed the conservative option with "watchful expectancy" or placing another chest tube and hoping for spontaneous resolution of the complication of the thoracic trauma mentioned in the previous paragraph. Thoracotomy, which was labeled as the most morbid of surgical incisions, was the only option when surgery became an absolute necessity

for the patient. The emergence of video-assisted thoracic surgery (VATS) in the early 1990s allowed surgeons access to the chest with lower morbidity. This approach may offer superior visualization, and a higher yield of detecting missed injuries. Unlike thoracotomy, the VATS approach is associated with less postoperative pain, better postoperative lung function, better postoperative shoulder function, shorter hospital stay, and in some cases reduced cost [8–13]. There have been some data to suggest that the immune function may be better preserved, the degree of inflammatory response less, and lung function better after VATS compared with thoracotomy, which benefits critically ill trauma patients [12,14,15].

The early series in which VATS was used for trauma applied it to the diagnosis of diaphragmatic injuries. Ochsner and coworkers [16] diagnosed nine diaphragmatic injuries in 14 patients by using this technique. Some of the current indications for VATS for trauma are listed in Table 1.

Management of retained hemothorax with video-assisted thoracic surgery

Hemothorax frequently occurs after chest trauma. Unfortunately, tube thoracostomy is not always a perfect solution for this problem because of incomplete evacuation of the blood. It is estimated that 18% to 30% of patients with a hemothorax progress to have a retained hemothorax [5,6]. Operative intervention is required in 40% of these patients because of persistent

* Corresponding author
  E-mail address: shazelrigg@siumed.edu
(S.R. Hazelrigg).

Table 1
Specific indications of video-assisted thoracic surgery in
thoracic trauma

Management of retained hemothorax
Management of persistent pneumothorax
Evaluation of diaphragm in penetrating
   thoracoabdominal injuries
Management of posttraumatic empyema
Management of ongoing bleeding in hemodynamically
   stable patients
Other rare indications: retrieval of foreign bodies,
   traumatic chylothorax, rib resections

hematoma or complications related to the hemothorax, such as empyema, respiratory insufficiency, or fibrothorax [5,17,18].

For years, the treatment for complicated
retained hemothorax had been thoracotomy and
drainage or decortication when complications
(empyema, trapped lung) occurred. Because of
the significant morbidity of thoracotomy, the
conservative route (chest tube drainage or
"watchful expectancy") for the spontaneous resolution had been a common approach. The delay
in a surgical decision resulted in a thicker fibrinous peel, more empyema, and an increase in
mortality and morbidity [17–19]. Advances in
minimally invasive surgery and the use of fibrinolytic agents have recently reformed the treatment
of retained hemothorax resulting in better outcomes [5,6,13,20–22]. The timing and threshold
for operative intervention shifted after VATS
emerged in the early 1990s.

In 1979, Wilson and coworkers [23] retrospectively reviewed 408 patients who had chest tube
drainage for a traumatic hemothorax. Two hundred ninety patients had complete resolution of
hemothorax at the time of chest tube removal
(Group 1A) and 118 had a residual hemothorax
(Group 1B). The incidence of long-term pleural
abnormality was 11% (Group 1A) and 16%
(Group 1B), and empyema was 4.8% and 5.1%,
respectively. The abnormal chest radiograph was
either treated with observation, chest tube, or
thoracentesis. Permanent changes in chest radiographs were often considered acceptable in the
1970s to the alternative of thoracotomy and decortication. In this group of patients, three ultimately underwent invasive thoracic procedures.
Eloesser flap (N = 2) and decortication of fibrous
peel (N = 1) were performed. Collins and coworkers [24], despite the morbidity of thoracotomy in 1978, compared the results of early

decortication for retained hemothorax with late
decortication in a small group of patients. They
found infectious complications and hospital stay
(6.1 days versus 9.8 days) were significantly improved in the early thoracotomy group. Coselli
and coworkers [19] reviewed 4000 patients who
were treated for hemothorax. One hundred fifty-
five (3.8%) needed thoracotomy. These patients
were divided into three groups: (1) early thoracotomy (within the first 5 days); (2) thoracotomy and
decortication after 5 days of admission; and (3)
thoracotomy for empyema as a complication of
retained hemothorax. No empyema and no mortality occurred among patients who were treated
early. The mortality was 1.6% and 9.4% in
groups 2 and 3, respectively. The hospital stay
was 10 days in the early group versus 37.9 days
in the late intervention groups. Eddy and coworkers [25] reviewed 117 patients who needed
thoracostomy for hemothorax or pneumothorax.
The rate of empyema is 10.2%, and 50% of
patients having a retained hemothorax.

The debate of early thoracotomy versus watchful expectancy for the spontaneous resolution of
retained hemothorax came to an end with the
widespread use of VATS. The addition of video
and indirect vision removed the awkward and
potentially nonsterile necessity for the surgeon's
head to be at the end of the telescope, provided
a panoramic view of the chest cavity, and allowed
assistants to observe and efficiently help during the
procedures. This resulted in the rapid adoption of
thoracoscopy. It has also been shown that VATS
has a lesser degree of pain, length of stay, and cost
compared with conventional thoracotomy.

Mancini and coworkers [20] first described the
use of VATS for the early evacuation of retained
clot after trauma. They reported three cases, of
which two were successfully treated with VATS
and one needed to be converted to a thoracotomy.
All three patients had penetrating injuries. The
first two patients were successfully operated on
within 48 hours of admission, whereas the third
patient was 7 days away from injury and had adhesions that required the conversion to thoracotomy. Subsequently, Heniford and coworkers [6]
reviewed a 25-patient series where four were converted to open thoracotomy. They found that the
patients who were treated successfully with VATS
were operated on within the first 7 days (mean =
4.5 days) of admission and they had a significantly
shorter hospital stay and no empyema was observed. The mean preoperative hospital stay for
patients who had an unsuccessful VATS was

14.5 days. Similarly, Amborgi and coworkers [26] had one conversion in 33 patients, and this patient was operated on over 10 days after admission. They found that the operating time, hospital stay, and postoperative days of chest tube duration were shorter in patients who were operated on within the first 7 days. In 39 months of follow-up there were no reaccumulations or persistent chest radiograph abnormalities.

Meyer and coworkers [13] prospectively evaluated patients with retained hemothoraces and randomized these patients to have a second chest tube (N = 24) or VATS (N = 15). The time of randomization was within the first 48 hours of hospital admission. Additional chest tube placement failed to resolve the problem in 10 of 24 patients, and these patients referred for either thoracotomy (N = 5) or VATS (N = 5). The length of hospital stay (3.6 versus 7.21 days after procedure) and cost of hospital stay ($7689 versus $13,273) was significantly lower in the patients who were originally enrolled in the VATS group. None of the patients who were originally assigned to the VATS group required conversion to thoracotomy and no mortality was recorded in any of the previously mentioned studies with a VATS approach.

The timing of VATS for retained hemothorax should be within the first 7 to 10 days [6,13,26]. A delay in intervention is associated with increased rate of conversion to thoracotomy. There is no clear indication for the amount of blood that necessitates evacuation, but recent literature has used 500 mL or symptoms as the threshold for VATS evacuation of blood [27,28]. The second attempt for a chest tube may be a suitable option for some patients, but overall results in increases in cost, hospital stay, and may increase the chance of requiring a thoracotomy [13].

Management of persistent retained pneumothorax and continued airleak with video-assisted thoracic surgery

Overall, the incidence of persistent pneumothorax with continuous airleak despite proper chest tube placement is about 4% to 23% after trauma [29,30]. Historically, this complication has been treated conservatively as long as it does not cause respiratory compromise or infection. Carillo [29] studied the use of VATS for persistent pneumothorax in 10 trauma patients. Chest tube management was an average of 10 days at the time of the VATS procedure. The duration of chest tube

after the stapling off of the injured part of lung was 48 hours. Nine of 10 patients were discharged from the hospital within 3 days. Schermer and coworkers [30] studied early VATS in patients who had an airleak after 3 days of admission. Thirtynine of 223 patients who required chest tubes for chest trauma qualified and were otherwise ready for discharge. They were randomized to two groups. Fourteen had conservative treatment and 25 had VATS repair. Four patients in the conservative group did have a delayed VATS. Total chest tube duration was 8.1 days versus 11.8 days and hospital stay was 9.7 versus 16.5 days, respectively. Surgery helped successfully identify and repair the source of leak in all but one patient. In that one patient, a mechanical pleurodesis was performed.

VATS is currently accepted as the standard of care for spontaneous pneumothorax. The recent literature suggests that this reduces the chest tube duration and hospital stay in patients with persistent posttraumatic pneumothorax [29,30]. It also allows the simultaneous detection of missed intrathoracic injuries, removal of foreign bodies, and removal of concomitant retained hemothorax. A preoperative detailed bronchoscopy should routinely be done to identify major airway injury. Shortening the need for chest tubes should reduce the incidence of serious hospital infections.

Use of video-assisted thoracic surgery in evaluation and treatment of traumatic diaphragm injuries

Diaphragmatic injuries have been more precisely diagnosed with the improvement of CT scanners and reconstruction software. In blunt trauma, CT is the preferred tool for the diagnosis of a diaphragmatic injury. For penetrating injuries, the diagnosis of the diaphragmatic injury remains a challenge. The incidence of diaphragmatic injuries is 20% to 59% with gunshot wounds and 15% to 32% with stab wounds in the thoracoabdominal region [5]. Unlike blunt injuries, the injuries caused by penetrating trauma are often small and clinical signs may initially be absent. Injuries to the diaphragm are important to diagnose because of concomitant intrathoracic and intra-abdominal injuries and the propensity for hernias to increase in size over time. Because of the negative pressure in the chest, organs and other contaminated contents may preferentially move into the thorax in patients with missed

diaphragmatic injuries, and this can lead to catastrophic complications. Peritoneal lavage for the
diagnosis of diaphragmatic injuries has had
a low yield and may cause serious respiratory
problems if the diaphragmatic injury exists and
there is no chest tube. Peritoneal lavage can be
used as an adjunct to rule out an associated intra-abdominal injury. It is possible to create a tension pneumothorax as a result of an attempt at
diagnostic laparoscopy. Even exploratory laparotomy can miss up to 15% of these injuries, especially when they are posterior [5].

VATS has been used for the diagnosis, and
sometimes repair, of diaphragmatic injuries for
more than a decade. Many of the early reports
about the use of VATS in thoracic trauma were
for the diagnosis of diaphragmatic injuries in
penetrating trauma [6,31]. In patients with thoracoabdominal trauma who do not have any abdominal injury and do not require laparotomy,
thoracoscopy is an excellent tool for the diagnosis and the treatment of diaphragmatic injury.
Ochsner and coworkers [16] investigated 14 patients with stab wounds and found that 9 of
the 14 thoracoscopies were positive for diaphragmatic injury. Freeman and coworkers [32] retrospectively reviewed patients who underwent
VATS after penetrating trauma to identify the
independent risk factors for diaphragmatic injury. The rate of diaphragmatic injury was 35%
in a total of 171 patients they reviewed. They
identified five risk factors that may suggest
a high probability of a diaphragmatic injury:
(1) abnormal chest radiograph in presentation,
(2) associated intra-abdominal trauma, (3) high-
velocity injuries, (4) entrance wound inferior to
the nipple or the scapula, and (5) a right-sided
entrance wound.

The accuracy of VATS is very high (98%–
100%) [16,30,32] in detecting a diaphragmatic injury and it allows removal of retained blood,
proper chest tube placement, repair of these injuries, and has no risk of tension pneumothorax.
This may reduce the chances of empyema in cases
where there is contamination of bile, or retained
hematoma, and also allows control of hemostasis
if there are any active bleeding sites. In cases
where there is an associated abdominal injury
that requires surgical repair, laparotomy has
been the approach of choice for repair of the
diaphragm.

The repair of the diaphragm should be done
with a suture technique because the stapling of the
diaphragm may result in late failure of the repair

because of the breakdown of the staple line
leading to later herniation.

The use of video-assisted thoracic surgery for posttraumatic empyema

In general, closed chest injuries are considered
sterile. Penetrating objects, such as chest tube
insertion, diaphragm rupture, hospital-acquired
pneumonia, atelectasis, impaired host defense
mechanisms caused by shock, contamination
through concomitant airleak, and massive blood
transfusions are contributing factors for infection.
Posttraumatic empyema is the third most frequent
cause of empyema after parapneumonic and postoperative etiologies. Among the intrathoracic
abnormalities created by trauma, hemothorax is
the leading cause of empyema [25]. Watkins and
coworkers [17] reviewed their blunt trauma patients who underwent decortications for empyema
in a 5-year period. They found that 23 of 28 patients who underwent surgery for empyema had
retained hemothorax-effusion. The retained blood
creates a perfect growth media for the bacteria.
The overall rate of empyema after hemothorax
ranges from 1.5% to 18% [4,17,25]. Empyema in
trauma patients may also occur in patients who
develop hospital-acquired pneumonia caused by
prolonged intubation and mechanical ventilation.

Normally, the acute or first phase of an
empyema lasts about 5 days. In this phase, the
fluid in the chest is thin and less cellular. The
second phase, or fibrinopurulent phase, occurs
between 5 and 21 days after injury. After this
time, VATS is generally technically not feasible
because of dense fibrinous peel that restricts
the lung. The success of VATS is close to 100%
in the early phases and the success rate falls in the
fibrinopurulent phase to 54% to 86%. The success
rate is indirectly proportional to time. After 3
weeks open decortication is necessary in most
cases [18,22]. In trauma, the time span for the formation of the fibrinous peel might even be shorter,
especially if there is contamination with blood, digestive tract contents, or bile. Timely evacuation
of residual blood and wash out of contamination
with thoracoscopy reduced empyema formation.
For the treatment of posttraumatic empyema,
VATS is recommended as the initial approach
for patients in the first two phases. A CT scan is
recommended before surgery to guide the initial
port placement and provide information about
the location of loculated fluid collections in the
chest.

Management of ongoing bleeding with video-assisted thoracic surgery

The indications for thoracic exploration for ongoing thoracic bleeding are well-defined in the trauma literature. Fifteen hundred milliliters of hemorrhagic drainage within the first hour of chest tube insertion or 200 to 300 mL/h drainage in subsequent 3 hours generally requires exploration.

For patients who are hemodynamically stable and do not fulfill the criteria for thoracotomy, VATS is an option for persistent bleeding. The approach allows the evacuation of any hematoma and the control of bleeding. In the few anecdotal reports on the use of VATS for this indication, bleeding is usually from intercostal or internal mammary injuries and injured lung segments [2,33,34]. The routine indication of exploratory VATS for ongoing bleeding is not well defined. There has been no prospective study to show its benefits; however, it can be used as an initial approach for patients who are hemodynamically stable but bleeding.

Other rare applications of video-assisted thoracic surgery after trauma

The use of VATS for intrathoracic foreign body removal is sparse in the literature. Most cases were for the removal of sponges and iatrogenic material. There are a small number of case reports for its use in trauma. It has been used for the retrieval of sharp objects, such as nails embedded by nail guns, stabbings, and pieces of large shrapnel. The goal has been to assess, repair the damage, and remove the sharp object in the controlled environment of the operating room with direct videoscopic observation of the thorax and mediastinum [35–37].

Traumatic chylothorax is rare. It may be created iatrogenically during the surgical repair of a left subclavian vessel, esophageal repair, or as a rare complication of insertion of a large-bore subclavian catheter. Primary injury to the thoracic duct or large thoracic lymphatics is extremely rare but may be associated with proximal clavicular fractures, or esophageal injuries. The first line of treatment is a combination of effective drainage and a low-fat diet, or nothing by mouth with total parenteral nutrition. Most traumatic chylothoraces close in 2 weeks with conservative management. If conservative treatment fails, however, the ligation of thoracic duct and pleurodesis is the surgical procedure of choice and can be performed with thoracoscopy.

Contraindications of video-assisted thoracic surgery in thoracic trauma

The general contraindications of VATS apply for trauma patients. Single-lung ventilation is preferred for VATS. Hence, patients who have significant pulmonary problems might not be good candidates for VATS. Adult respiratory distress syndrome and severe pulmonary contusion, which are not uncommon in trauma patients, may be contraindications for single-lung ventilation. Severe adhesions caused by prior surgeries are considered as a contraindication for VATS procedures. People who have had a prior decortication or chemical pleurodesis are not good candidates for VATS. Prior thoracoscopy and thoracotomy, however, are no longer considered as contraindications. The only reliable way to assess the adhesions and feasibility for VATS is observation of the chest with the videothoracoscope through a carefully created camera port at the beginning of the procedure. The authors generally place the first port away from any prior incision or chest tube sites to avoid likely areas of adhesions.

Any indication that mandates an emergency thoracotomy is obviously a contraindication for VATS. Hemodynamically unstable patients with chest injuries should undergo either urgent sternotomy or thoracotomy.

Technical note

After proper intubation with a double-lumen endotracheal tube, the patient is place in the full lateral decubitus position. If there are no trauma-related contraindications, the operating room table should be flexed to allow maximal separation of the ribs. This maneuver makes digital examination of the lung easier by increasing the intercostal distance, and it reduces the amount of trauma to intercostal nerves. Bronchoscopy should be done before every VATS to confirm the placement of a double-lumen endotracheal tube and also to rule out any major tracheobronchial injury.

The authors use a zero-degree lens for most VATS procedures but, based on the location and angle of the operating field, other angles can be used. The choice of trocar and camera size is based on the complexity of the surgery. Five-millimeter camera and ports can be used for simple procedures like pleural effusions and evacuation of simple hemothoraces. Up to 7% of patients who undergo VATS experience chronic intercostal nerve injury caused by the trauma of the camera or instrument ports. Using smaller size ports, flexing the table, and placement of trocars as anterior as possible are maneuvers that may help avoid the risk of intercostal nerve injury. The number and location of port sites are determined based on the complexity of surgery and location of the lesion. The trocars should be placed far enough apart to avoid "sword fights" during the procedure and always attempt to have all instruments move in the same direction. In thin patients, trocars can be avoided and instruments may be passed directly through incisions. The lung is handled with an atraumatic instrument, like a Duval clamp or ring forceps. Ring forceps and suction can be used to extract clot or fibrinopurulent exudate from the thorax. A power irrigator with suction can be used for a retained hemothorax or empyema surgery. Thoracotomy is always an available and appropriate option, and conversion is not a technical failure but often a sign of good judgment.

Summary

VATS is a valuable and safe way to manage many problems in thoracic trauma. It may allow earlier diagnosis and treatment of posttraumatic complications of chest injuries with less morbidity. This approach has already demonstrated advantages in such entities as retained hemothorax. The reduced pain and morbidity are attractive features compared with open thoracotomy. VATS continues to evolve in thoracic trauma, but unquestionably has proved value.

References

[1] Abolhoda A, Livingston DH, Donahoo JS, et al. Diagnostic and therapeutic video assisted thoracic surgery (VATS) following chest trauma. Eur J Cardiothorac Surg 1997;12:356–60.

[2] Manlulu AV, Lee TW, Thung KH, et al. Current indications and results of VATS in the evaluation and management of hemodynamically stable thoracic injuries. Eur J Cardiothorac Surg 2004;25:1048–53.

[3] Prabhakar G, Graeber G. Chest trauma: minimal access cardiothoracic surgery. In: Yim APC, Hazelrigg SR, Izzat MB, et al, editors. London: WB Saunders; 2000. p. 308–15.

[4] Mattox KL, Wall MJ, Pickard LR. Thoracic trauma. In: Feliciano D, Moore E, Mattox KL, editors. Trauma. 3rd edition. Stanford (CT): Appleton & Lang; 1996. p. 345–54.

[5] Ahmed N, Jones D. Video-assisted thoracic surgery: state of the art in trauma care. Int J Care Injured 2004;35:479–89.

[6] Heniford BT, Carrillo EH, Spain DA, et al. The role of thoracoscopy in the management of retained thoracic collections after trauma. Ann Thorac Surg 1997;63:940–3.

[7] Helling TS, Gyle NR, Einenstein CL. Complications following blunt and penetrating injuries in 216 victims of chest trauma requiring tube thoracostomy. J Trauma 1989;29:1367–70.

[8] Hazelrigg SR, Nunchuck SK, Landreneau RJ, et al. Cost analysis for thoracoscopy: thoracoscopic wedge resection. Ann Thorac Surg 1993;56(3): 633–5.

[9] Landreneau RJ, Hazelrigg SR, Mack MJ, et al. Postoperative pain-related morbidity: video-assisted thoracic surgery versus thoracotomy. Ann Thorac Surg 1993;56(6):1285–9.

[10] Landreneau RJ, Mack MJ, Hazelrigg SR, et al. Prevalence of chronic pain after pulmonary resection by thoracotomy or video-assisted thoracic surgery. J Thorac Cardiovasc Surg 1994;107(4): 1079–86.

[11] Hazelrigg SR, Cetindag IB, Fullerton J. Acute and chronic pain syndromes after thoracic surgery. Surg Clin North Am 2002;82(4):849–65.

[12] Cetindag IB, Olson W, Hazelrigg SR. Acute and chronic reduction of pulmonary function after lung surgery. Thorac Surg Clin 2004;14(3):317–23.

[13] Meyer DM, Jessen ME, Wait MA, et al. Early evacuation of traumatic retained hemothoraces using thoracoscopy: a prospective, randomized trial. Ann Thorac Surg 1997;64:1396–401.

[14] Craig SR, Leaver HA, Yap PL, et al. Acute phase responses following minimal access and conventional thoracic surgery. Eur J Cardiothorac Surg 2001; 20(3):455–63.

[15] Leaver HA, Craig SR, Yap PL, et al. Lymphocyte responses following open and minimally invasive thoracic surgery. Eur J Clin Invest 2000;30(3):230–8.

[16] Ochsner MG, Rozycki GS, Lucente F, et al. Prospective evaluation of thoracoscopy for diagnosing diaphragmatic injury in thoracoabdominal trauma: a preliminary report. J Trauma 1993;34(5):704–10.

[17] Watkins JA, Spain DA, Richardson JD, et al. Empyema and restrictive pleural processes after blunt trauma: an under-recognized cause of respiratory failure. Am Surg 2000;66(2):210–4.

[18] Mandal AK, Thadepalli H, Mandal AK, et al. Posttraumatic empyema thoracis: a 24-year experience at a major trauma center. J Trauma 1997;43(5):764–71.

[19] Coselli JS, Mattox KL, Beall AC Jr. Reevaluation of early evacuation of clotted hemothorax. Am J Surg 1984;148(6):786–90.

[20] Mancini M, Smith LM, Nein A, et al. Early evacuation of clotted blood in hemothorax using thoracoscopy: case reports. J Trauma 1993;34(1):144–7.

[21] Inci I, Ozcelik C, Ulku R, et al. Intrapleural fibrinolytic treatment of traumatic clotted hemothorax. Chest 1998;114:160–5.

[22] Landreneau RJ, Keenan RJ, Hazelrigg SR, et al. Thoracoscopy for empyema and hemothorax. Chest 1996;109(1):18–24.

[23] Wilson JM, Boren CH Jr, Peterson SR, et al. Traumatic hemothorax: is decortication necessary? J Thorac Cardiovasc Surg 1979;77:489–95.

[24] Collins MP, Shuck JM, Wachtel TL, et al. Early decortication after thoracic trauma. Arch Surg 1978; 113(4):440–5.

[25] Eddy AC, Luna GK, Copass M. Empyema thoracis in patients undergoing emergent closed tube thoracostomy for thoracic trauma. Am J Surg 1989; 157(5):494–7.

[26] Ambrogi MC, Lucchi M, Dini P, et al. Videothoracoscopy for evaluation and treatment of hemothorax. J Cardiovasc Surg (Torino) 2002;43(1):109–12.

[27] Velmahos GC, Demetriades D. Early thoracoscopy for the evacuation of undrained haemothorax. Eur J Surg 1999;165:924–9.

[28] Carrillo EH, Richardson JD. Thoracoscopy for the acutely injured patient. Am J Surg 2005;190:234–8.

[29] Carrillo EH, Schmacht DC, Gable DR, et al. Thoracoscopy in the management of posttraumatic persistent pneumothorax. J Am Coll Surg 1998;186(6): 636–40.

[30] Schermer CR, Matteson BD, Demarest GB 3rd, et al. A prospective evaluation of video-assisted thoracic surgery for persistent air leak due to trauma. Am J Surg 1999;177(6):480–4.

[31] Jackson AM, Ferreira AA. Thoracoscopy as an aid to the diagnosis of diaphragmatic injury in penetrating wounds of the left lower chest: a preliminary report. Injury 1976;7(3):213–7.

[32] Freeman RK, Al-Dossari G, Hutcheson KA, et al. Indications for using video-assisted thoracoscopic surgery to diagnose diaphragmatic injuries after penetrating chest trauma. Ann Thorac Surg 2001; 72(2):342–7.

[33] Pons F, Lang-Lazdunski L, deKerangal X, et al. The role of videothoracoscopy in management of precordial thoracic penetrating injuries. Eur J Cardiothorac Surg 2002;22(1):7–12.

[34] Smith RS, Fry WR, Tsoi EK, et al. Preliminary report on videothoracoscopy in the evaluation and treatment of thoracic injury. Am J Surg 1993; 166(6):690–5.

[35] Williams CG, Haut ER, Ouyang H, et al. Video-assisted thoracic surgery removal of foreign bodies after penetrating chest trauma. J Am Coll Surg 2006;202(5):848–52.

[36] Hanvesakul R, Momin A, Gee MJ, et al. A role for video assisted thoracoscopy in stable penetrating chest trauma. Emerg Med J 2005;22(5):386–7.

[37] Lang-Lazdunski L, Mouroux J, Pons F, et al. Role of videothoracoscopy in chest trauma. Ann Thorac Surg 1997;63(2):327–33.

ELSEVIER
SAUNDERS

Thorac Surg Clin 17 (2007) 81–85

THORACIC
SURGERY
CLINICS

Traumatic Diaphragmatic Injuries

James R. Scharff, MD, Keith S. Naunheim, MD*

St. Louis University Medical Center, 3635 Vista Avenue, St. Louis, MO 63110–0250, USA

Traumatic diaphragmatic hernias are classified both with regard to etiology and with regard to the time of presentation. Both of these factors may have a significant effect not only on the signs and symptoms of presentation but also on the optimal method for diagnostic evaluation and surgical therapy.

The etiology includes traumatic diaphragmatic hernias from blunt trauma, penetrating trauma, and iatrogenic injury. Blunt trauma most commonly occurs secondary to motor vehicle accidents or falls from a height. Although the exact pathophysiologic mechanism is uncertain, Kearney and coworkers [1] has postulated that a direct anterior blow to the abdomen may significantly increase intra-abdominal pressure and exceed the bursting pressure of the diaphragm itself. He also proposed that a lateral blow can cause sheer force, which may result in detachment of the diaphragm from its insertion on the chest wall. Recent work by Reiff and coworkers [2] has suggested that obesity may play a role in such injuries. His analysis of a national automotive database sought to identify independent risk factors for diaphragmatic rupture following all types of motor vehicle collisions. Reiff noted that although an elevated body mass index of greater than or equal to 30 was not significantly associated with diaphragmatic injury overall, an elevated body mass index did seem to be an increased risk factor for such injury in patient's with near side motor vehicle collisions as opposed to those involved in head-on accidents.

The pathophysiology of penetrating trauma is not as uncertain as that of blunt trauma. Both stab wounds and gunshot wounds can cause diaphragmatic lacerations and do result in injury to the diaphragm more often than does blunt trauma. A gunshot wound virtually anywhere within the chest or abdomen puts the patient at risk for penetrating diaphragmatic trauma because of the projectile's potentially prolonged length of travel within the body. For stab wounds, however, the limited length of a blade (usually 8 in or less) suggests that a stab wound needs to be within 6 to 8 in of the extent of diaphragmatic excursion if it is to cause a penetrating injury. Stab wounds at or below the level of the nipple and above the umbilicus are the only ones that are at risk for causing such damage.

Iatrogenic injuries to the diaphragm may occur either during open abdominal or thoracic procedures. They can also be more insidious, however, such as diaphragmatic laceration during thoracentesis or secondary to radiofrequency ablation [3]. Such injuries can be difficult to identify because of a low index of suspicion.

Incidence

Diaphragmatic injuries appear in 1% to 7% of patients with significant blunt trauma and in 10% to 15% of those with penetrating wounds [4–6]. Although autopsy studies suggest an equal incidence of diaphragmatic lacerations on the left and right, in the clinical world left-sided lesions predominate with recognized right-sided diaphragmatic occurring only between one half [7,8] to one third [9] as often. This may be because of a cushioning or buffering effect of the liver on the right side. Bilateral lacerations are relatively rare and occur in 1% to 2% of patients [9].

Left-sided defects may present with herniation of the stomach, large bowel, small bowel, spleen,

* Corresponding author.
  E-mail address: naunheim@slu.edu
  (K.S. Naunheim).

liver, or omentum. Right-sided perforations generally are limited to protrusion of the liver, large bowel, or omentum into the thoracic cavity. Right-sided diaphragmatic rupture may also occasionally be associated with significant vascular tears in the inferior vena cava or hepatic vein, lesions that are particularly morbid.

Clinical presentation

A history of trauma is always obtainable, although in cases of chronic herniation this may require persistent and detailed questioning regarding prior medical history. A high index of clinical suspicion is likely the clinician's best tool when seeking to make the diagnosis of traumatic perforation. Very often there is no sign or symptom directly attributable to the diaphragmatic defect. Most commonly symptoms are secondary to concomitant injuries, which occur quite frequently. Serious central nervous system injury occurs in 10% to 20% of patients, cardiothoracic injuries in 20% to 60% of patients, musculoskeletal problems in 30% to 40%, and intra-abdominal injuries in 60% to 100% of patients [6]. Often, signs and symptoms of these concomitant injuries mask the clinical picture and prevent initial suspicion of a diaphragmatic injury. Symptoms that may be referable to diaphragmatic injury include shoulder pain, epigastric pain, respiratory distress, and intrathoracic bowel sounds in patients with acute diaphragmatic injury. The diagnosis occasionally comes to light in less standard fashion. On occasion intrathoracic bowel may be palpated during placement of a chest tube or bilious fluid may be seen exiting from a previously placed chest tube.

In patients with delayed presentation, symptomatology of partial or complete intestinal obstruction predominates. Pain typically occurs in the epigastric area or in either upper quadrant. It may worsen with meals and be associated with nausea or vomiting. When this recurs chronically in a subacute fashion it can be mistaken for peptic ulcer disease, cholecystitis, or pancreatitis. The pain may occasionally radiate to the left shoulder, a symptom that can be mistaken for myocardial ischemia secondary to coronary artery disease.

When intestinal obstruction occurs as a result of an incarcerated intrathoracic length of bowel, the symptoms and physical findings depend on the anatomic level of obstruction. Gastric herniation through the left diaphragm causes signs and symptoms much like those of gastric volvulus secondary to paraesophageal herniation. An inability to swallow associated with retching and regurgitation of foamy saliva may be the most prominent signs and symptoms. In such a case the abdomen is likely nondistended and quiet. Cases in which the colon or distal small bowel have herniated into the left chest, however, present with more classic signs of intestinal obstruction including abdominal distention, tympany, and hyperactive bowel sounds.

In those rare occasions when a complete closed loop obstruction occurs within the chest, massive distention of the viscus can occur and may cause shortness of breath and cyanosis caused by mediastinal shift and pulmonary compression.

Diagnosis

There is rarely anything specific or definitive from the clinical history or physical examination that points the clinician toward diagnosis of diaphragmatic rupture. Once again, high index of suspicion is likely the most important attribute that allows for an early diagnosis.

The chest radiograph is usually the first hint regarding the possibility of diaphragmatic injury. Intrathoracic air in a silhouette consistent with supradiaphragmatic viscera may occur in up to 50% of patients with left-sided diaphragmatic herniation. The identification of a nasogastric tube passing first to an infradiaphragmatic position and then upward into the chest is pathognomonic for gastric herniation. In patients with right-sided diaphragmatic injury, an elevated diaphragm is often initially diagnosed until it is recognize that the liver has herniated into the chest. Colonic herniation through a right-sided defect can also be seen.

Often, however, the chest radiograph is obscured by the presence of fluid or hemothorax or lung contusion. In such cases a chest CT scan can be diagnostic [6,10,11]. Axial CT views of the chest and abdomen often allow for a diagnosis to be made but, on occasion, three-dimensional reconstruction with sagittal and coronal views may also be helpful. Modern technology using multidetector scanners allows for diagnostic precision, often allowing for identification and exact localization of the diaphragmatic defect.

Other potential methods of diagnosis include ultrasound and magnetic resonance imaging of the chest or abdomen. Both of these have only limited use in patients with acute herniation, whereas both chest radiograph and CT scan are routinely performed in such patients to assess the extent of injury. Contrast studies, such as barium enema or barium swallow, may be helpful when there is suspicion of intrathoracic herniation. The typical appearance is that of a loop of large bowel or small bowel within the chest with a "pinch" or narrow "neck" at the level of the diaphragm (Fig. 1). In the distant past, diagnostic pneumoperitoneum or the intraperitoneal injection of technetium had been used to identify the presence of connection between the abdominal and thoracic cavities. Neither is required given present technology.

In the case of penetrating trauma it is possible for a diaphragmatic injury to occur without the immediate herniation of intra-abdominal contents within the chest. Because of the extant pressure gradient across such a defect (positive intra-abdominal pressure and negative intrathoracic pressure) a herniation of intra-abdominal structures into the chest may occur over time, leading to delayed presentation. Such lesions occur more frequently secondary to stab wounds than they do with gunshot wounds and they can be exceedingly difficult to diagnose. In such cases chest radiograph, chest CT scan, and all contrast studies are nondiagnostic in the acute setting. When there remains a high index of suspicion regarding the potential for diaphragmatic injury, however, direct visualization either by laparoscopy [12,13] or thoracoscopy [14,15] may be undertaken to allow

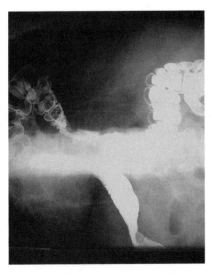

Fig. 1. Anterior diaphragmatic rupture allowing intrathoracic protrusion of transverse colon. Note "pinch" at the level of the diaphragmatic defect.

direct visualization of the diaphragm and exclusion of a diaphragmatic defect. In this fashion, minimally invasive procedures can be useful for the early identification and repair of small diaphragmatic lesions and may prevent delayed presentation with potentially catastrophic results.

Treatment

Because of the risk for intestinal obstruction and visceral strangulation, the identification of any diaphragmatic defect is in itself adequate indication for surgical repair. Many such patients, however, present with concomitant injuries or hypovolemic shock and attention must first be paid to resuscitation and treatment of more immediately life-threatening lesions, such as hemothorax, hemopericardium, splenic or hepatic lacerations, and vascular injuries. Often the presence of such lesions dictates whether the initial exploration is undertaken through a thoracotomy or a laparotomy. Although the diaphragm can be adequately repaired through either transthoracic or transabdominal approach, there are certain situations in which one approach is preferable to the other.

Surgical dogma suggests that in cases of acute herniation secondary to abdominal trauma, laparotomy provides the best mode of diaphragmatic repair. It allows for concomitant treatment of any intra-abdominal injuries, and the reduction of acutely herniated viscera is easily undertaken from this approach. If, during laparotomy, it is recognized that there is significant injury to the inferior vena cava or the hepatic veins, it may be best to extend an incision upward and perform an urgent median sternotomy. In this fashion one can gain control of the inferior vena cava and potentially use a temporary shunt to effect repairs [7].

For those patient's who have significant hemothorax with continuing output of blood from a chest tube, a thoracotomy approach is likely indicated and the diaphragm can easily be repaired through this approach. The patients in whom both significant intra-abdominal and intrathoracic bleeding occur can be treated with a thoracoabdominal approach, although this somewhat increases the morbidity of the procedure.

In the acute situation with an absence of signs of intra-abdominal damage or hemorrhage, a right thoracic approach is often the best choice for right-sided diaphragmatic rupture. A right-sided diaphragm repair from an intra-abdominal approach can be difficult because of the bulk of the liver, which may obscure the posterior edge of diaphragmatic defect. A supradiaphragmatic approach often proves far easier on the right and is likely the approach of choice.

For patients in whom delayed rupture is identified, a thoracic approach is often considered to be optimal. The presence of abdominal viscera in the chest often leads to significant adhesions to intrathoracic structures and these can be difficult to take down from an abdominal approach. A thoracotomy with intrathoracic dissection and subsequent diaphragmatic repair is the approach of choice.

There have been several reports of a laparoscopic approach for the management of chronic traumatic or diaphragmatic hernias. Shaw and coworkers [16] reported the use of a laparoscopic-assisted approach using a 4- to 5-cm subcostal incision with traction on the abdominal wall. A more traditional laparoscopic approach was reported by Matthews and colleagues [17] who were able to repair 13 of 17 such diaphragmatic defects through a laparoscopic approach. Most cases that were converted to laparotomy occurred because of the difficulty in repairing central lesions immediately adjacent to or underneath the pericardium.

Although it is certainly possible to approach chronic diaphragmatic hernias with minimally invasive techniques through either laparoscopy or thoracoscopy, such procedures require advanced training and experience and are not likely appropriate for most surgeons. In the acute setting in patients with serious concomitant injuries, an open operative approach is indicated.

The method of repair reported has been highly variable and it is hard to identify a gold standard. A direct repair is usually possible and routine use of a prosthetic graft is discouraged. In chronic diaphragmatic hernias it may be necessary to enlarge the diaphragmatic opening and if one does so this extension of the defect should be undertaken radially in a direction away from the central tendon so as to avoid division of phrenic nerve branches with resultant diaphragmatic dysfunction. For cases in which the hernia is identified months to years after the initial injury there may be sufficient scarring and tissue retraction that primary closure becomes difficult or impossible. In such cases, closure using an occlusive prosthetic material, such as a thick polytetrafluoroethylene graft, can be undertaken. Although biologic materials have also been suggested for

grafts in such cases, such materials are more expensive and seem to yield little clinical advantage.

When one undertakes a direct closure, it can be achieved with a number of suture techniques. The authors' method of repair entails using interrupted horizontal mattress sutures of 0 braided nylon. Both one and two layer closures have been described, however, using simple sutures, figure-of-eight sutures, running suture lines, or a combination of these suture techniques. Although there is no single correct technique of closure, the principles for repair include complete reduction of the viscera, watertight closure with nonabsorbable suture, and minimizing any additional injury to phrenic innervation of the diaphragm.

On occasion, one finds a diaphragmatic detachment from the chest wall. In such cases resuspension may be undertaken to reattach the diaphragm to the chest wall. The authors' preferred technique includes use of nonabsorbable horizontal mattress sutures placed full thickness through the diaphragm and through the entire chest wall, with the sutures being tied in the submuscular space on the outside of the chest wall.

Outcome

The mortality for diaphragmatic repairs is generally dictated by the number and severity of concomitant injuries. There is a wide variation in mortality results for diaphragmatic herniation secondary to both blunt trauma (15%–40%) and penetrating trauma (10%–30%) [6,9]. A recent multivariate analysis looked at clinical factors in 731 patients with traumatic diaphragmatic hernias to identify predictors of mortality [8]. The investigators identified three independent predictors including an elevated injury severity score, transfusion requirement of greater than 10 units of packed red blood cells, and the need for urgent thoracotomy. Not surprisingly, all three factors portend a poor outcome.

In cases of chronic herniation in which there are no concomitant injuries requiring repair, the mortality is determined by the presence of patient comorbidities, such as cardiac arrhythmias, coronary artery disease, chronic pulmonary disease, and renal insufficiency. In the absence of such serious medical problems the mortality should approach that of exploratory thoracotomy with simple repair of a lung injury.

Summary

Although numerous articles have been written over the past two decades with regard to the treatment of traumatic diaphragmatic hernia, little has actually changed during that time. The ability to make the diagnosis has somewhat improved because of the technologic advances in CT; however, it remains true that the best tool to guide the clinician toward the appropriate diagnosis is a high index of suspicion in patients with blunt or appropriate penetrating trauma. Although laparoscopic or thoracoscopic management of such patients may become prevalent with increasing experience, at present the open approach and simple repair remain the mainstays of management. The patient's survival still depends more on the severity of concomitant nondiaphragmatic injuries and in many cases the diaphragmatic laceration is the least worrisome and least morbid of the patient's injuries. Operative repair results in a good outcome in most patients in the absence of other serious injuries.

References

[1] Kearney PA, Rouhana SW, Burney RE. Blunt rupture of the diaphragm: mechanism, diagnosis, and treatment. Ann of Emerg Med 1989;18:1326–30.

[2] Reiff DA, Davis RP, MacLennan PA, et al. The association between body mass index and diaphragm injury among motor vehicle collision occupants. J Trauma 2004;57:1324–8.

[3] Koda M, Ueki M, Maeda N, et al. Diaphragmatic perforation and hernia after hepatic radiofrequency ablation. AJR Am J Roentgenol 2003;180:1561–2.

[4] Boulanger BR, Mirvis SE, Rodriguez A. Magnetic resonance imaging in traumatic diaphragmatic rupture: case reports. J Trauma 1992;32:89–93.

[5] Sarna S, Kivioja A. Blunt rupture of the diaphragm. Ann Chir Gynaecol 1995;84:261–5.

[6] Rosati C. Acute traumatic injury of the diaphragm. Chest Surg Clin N Am 1998;8:371–9.

[7] Estrera AS, Landay MJ, McClelland RN. Blunt traumatic rupture of the right hemidiaphragm: experience in 12 patients. Ann Thorac Surg 1985;39: 525–30.

[8] Williams M, Carlin AM, Tyburski JG, et al. Predictors of mortality in patients with traumatic diaphragmatic rupture and associated thoracic and/or abdominal injuries. Am Surg 2004;70:157–62.

[9] Shah R, Sabanathan S, Mearns AJ, et al. Traumatic rupture of diaphragm. Ann Thorac Surg 1995;60: 1444–9.

[10] Marts B, Durham R, Shapiro M, et al. Computed tomography in the diagnosis of blunt thoracic injury. Am J Surg 1994;168:688–92.

[11] Sliker CW. Imaging of diaphragm injuries. Radiol Clin North Am 2006;44:199–211.

[12] Ivatury RR. The role of laparoscopy in establishing diaphragmatic injury in lower chest wounds. J Trauma 2005;58:1305–10.

[13] Friese RS, Coln CE, Gentilello LM. Laparoscopy is sufficient to exclude occult diaphragm injury after penetrating abdominal trauma. J Trauma 2005;58: 789–92.

[14] Lowdermilk GA, Naunheim KS. Thoracoscopic evaluation and treatment of thoracic trauma. Surg Clin N Am 2000;80:1535–42.

[15] Freeman RK, Al-Dossari G, Hutcheson KA, et al. Indications for using video-assisted thoracoscopic surgery to diagnose diaphragmatic injuries after penetrating chest trauma. Ann Thorac Surg 2001; 72:342–7.

[16] Shaw JM, Navsaria PH, Nicol AJ. Laparoscopy-assisted repair of diaphragm injuries. World J Surg 2003;27:671–4.

[17] Matthews BD, Bui H, Harold KL, et al. Laparoscopic repair of traumatic diaphragmatic injuries. Surg Endosc 2003;17:254–8.

ELSEVIER
SAUNDERS

Thorac Surg Clin 17 (2007) 87–93

THORACIC
SURGERY
CLINICS

Cardiac Trauma

Richard Embrey, MD

*Department of Surgery, Southern Illinois University School of Medicine, P.O. Box 19638,
Springfield, IL 62794–19638, USA*

Fifty years ago, nearly all significant cardiac injuries were fatal, many were untreatable, and most were undiagnosed until the autopsy suite. In the last 20 years, however, dramatic improvements in prehospital trauma management, new diagnostic modalities, and the availability of cardiac surgery in many hospitals have rendered treatable most cardiac injuries. Knowledge of various types of cardiac injuries, the methods available to facilitate rapid diagnosis, and familiarity with techniques for surgical repair are no longer an academic exercise but a lifesaving necessity.

Blunt cardiac injuries

Cardiac injuries occur in up to 30% of blunt trauma patients [1,2]. The mechanism of such injuries includes direct precordial impact, compression of the chest with abrupt increase in intrathoracic pressure, high-speed deceleration, or a combination of more than one type. The most common cause of blunt cardiac injury is motor vehicle accident, but it can occur in the setting of industrial accidents, falls, and even with a seemingly innocuous sports injury or animal kick.

Pericardial rupture

Tears in the pericardium are rare, and even more rarely diagnosed. Because pericardial injury is often seen in connection with myocardial contusion or rupture of the heart, the pathophysiology of injury is likely the same: high-energy precordial impact or a hydraulic mechanism, such as sudden increase in intrabdominal pressure [3]. The most common site for tears is parallel to the left phrenic nerve (64%), along the diaphragmatic surface (18%) and parallel

to the right phrenic nerve (18%) [4]. Small tears are of no consequence, but larger tears can lead to herniation of the heart and dramatic compromise of systemic venous return [5]. Chest roentgenography is often highly suggestive of the diagnosis of pericardial rupture, with obvious lateral displacement of the heart into either chest (Fig. 1) or bowel gas in the pericardial sac. Other diagnostic tests, such as CT scan and echocardiography, are often not very helpful. If cardiac compromise because of pericardial rupture is suspected, sternotomy or thoracotomy and repair of the defect should be undertaken.

Commotio cordis

Sudden cardiac death from seemingly modest blows to the anterior chest is a rare but horrifying consequence of competitive and recreational sports. Occurring primarily in males (95%) and in adolescents or children (78%), commotio cordis is caused by a sharp blow to the precordium during the vulnerable phase of repolarization (just before T-wave peak), resulting in ventricular fibrillation or asystole [6]. These lethal arrhythmias can result from being struck by baseballs, softballs, hockey pucks, fists, and even plastic bats. Protective padding is not assurance of complete safety. Only 13% of victims survive commotio cordis, and survival is directly correlated with quick recognition, rapid initiation of resuscitation, and the availability of automatic external defibrillators in gymnasia and sports complexes.

Myocardial contusion

Myocardial contusion is the most common blunt cardiac injury, occurring in 14% of fatal blunt trauma patients [7]. It can be frequently overlooked, however, when other more obvious

E-mail address: rembrey@siumed.edu

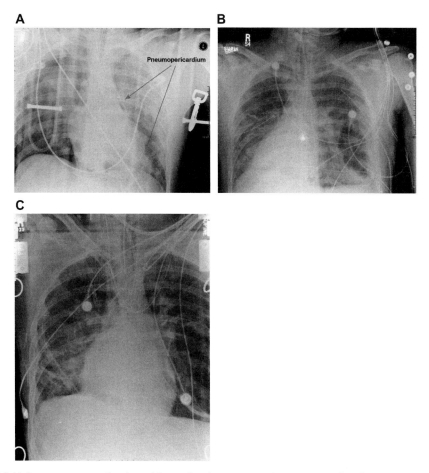

Fig. 1. (A) Initial roentgenogram of patient with massive chest trauma. Note pneumopericardium and right pneumothorax. (B) Subsequent chest radiograph of the same patient. Note displacement of cardiac silhouette into the right chest. (C) Postoperative of patient following repair of pericardial tear caused by blunt trauma.

and urgent injuries are present. Unfortunately, myocardial contusion is a somewhat vague term and is applied to the entire spectrum of blunt myocardial injury, ranging from myocardial stunning without demonstrable myocyte damage to transmural necrosis and hemorrhage [8]. As such, the term is attached to both patients with uncomplicated cardiac enzyme elaboration and to those who succumb to ventricular rupture.

Patients suffering from myocardial contusion caused by blunt trauma may be viewed as analogous to those suffering ischemic myocardial infarctions. Many cases of myocardial contusion are limited and uncomplicated (ie, non–ST-segment elevation myocardial infarctions), but a few lead to life-threatening sequelae, such as arrhythmia, low cardiac output, ventricular rupture, and atrioventricular valve regurgitation caused by

papillary muscle necrosis (transmural infarction). Evaluation and management of patients with myocardial contusion parallels that of myocardial infarction.

The clinical diagnosis of myocardial contusion can be complex, and no single test is perfectly sensitive or completely predictive of complications. An ECG and cardiac troponin I should be obtained in all patients admitted to the emergency department with blunt force trauma to the thorax or upper abdomen and a second cardiac troponin I level obtained at 6 hours following admission. If the patient remains asymptomatic and cardiac troponin I is below 1.05 μg/L, then myocardial contusion can be reasonably excluded [9]. If either is abnormal, then the patient should receive serial cardiac troponin I determinations and continuous cardiac monitoring for 48 hours.

Myocardial contusion should be suspected in any patient with significant chest trauma and unexplained hypotension despite volume resuscitation. Central venous and arterial pressure monitoring can be indispensable in making a diagnosis of myocardial dysfunction caused by contusion [10]. Transesophageal echocardiography has proved very useful in confirming the presence of ventricular dysfunction in patients with suspected myocardial contusion [11]. MRI and positron emission tomography have both been used to determine myocardial viability in cardiac contusion, but have limited clinical usefulness [12,13].

Treatment of patients with symptomatic myocardial contusion is primarily supportive. Inotropes can be very effective in maintaining arterial pressure and cardiac output. Arrhythmias should be anticipated and can be controlled pharmacologically; occasionally, temporary transvenous cardiac pacing is required for the rare instance of high-grade atrioventricular block following myocardial contusion. Intra-aortic balloon counterpulsation has been used successfully in a handful of cases.

Severe, transmural myocardial contusion may lead to any of several complications similar to those seen with ischemic myocardial infarction, such as delayed ventricular rupture, ventricular aneurysm formation, ventricular septal defect, and papillary muscle rupture. These complications can occur anywhere from hours to weeks following injury, and patients with severe myocardial contusion should be closely monitored for up to a month [14].

Cardiac valve injury

Cardiac valve injury is a rare complication of blunt chest trauma. The mechanism of injury is a sudden increase in intravascular or intracardiac pressure while the valve is closed [15]. For the aortic valve (the most commonly injured) this is in early diastole, when a tremendous pressure gradient can be developed across the closed valve with sudden, severe compression of the chest. The atrioventricular valves are most susceptible to injury when the trauma occurs in late diastole or early systole when the maximally dilated ventricles tense the subvalvular apparatus [16].

The diagnosis of traumatic valve injury should be entertained by the presence of a cardiac murmur or onset of congestive heart failure. The clinical symptoms may vary widely, from none to cardiogenic shock. Echocardiography is indicated

when the diagnosis of traumatic valve injury is suspected. Cardiac catheterization is not required, except in patients where coronary angiography is warranted before cardiac surgery.

Often, the damaged valves can be repaired, depending on the extent of damage. Isolated avulsion of the noncoronary cusp of the aortic valve is amenable to resuspension, although the long-term durability of the repair is uncertain. Many surgeons are facile with mitral and tricuspid repair techniques, such as replacement of ruptured chordae and patching of annular tears. When papillary muscle rupture is present, however, mitral valve replacement may be necessary in critically ill patients [17].

Coronary artery injuries

Coronary artery injury is exceedingly rare, occurring in less than 2% of cases of blunt chest trauma [18]. Most coronary injuries are characterized by intimal tears leading to dissection and frequently to thrombosis (Fig. 2). Complete or partial transection of the coronary at its origin from the aorta can also occur. Mechanism of injury is most often rapid deceleration (motor vehicle accidents and falls), although coronary dissection after low-energy blows to the chest can occur.

Not surprisingly, coronary artery injury often appears as an acute myocardial infarction with ST-segment elevation in ECG leads corresponding to the involved coronary artery. Hypotension and ventricular arrhythmias are common. Coronary

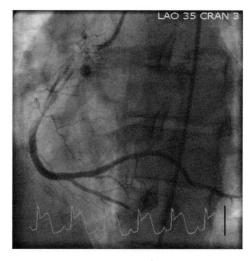

Fig. 2. Right coronary angiogram of patient with intimal flap following motor vehicle accident leading to inferior wall myocardial infarction.

transection or intrapericardial rupture of a dissected artery produces tamponade. It is important to be aware that these signs and symptoms may not develop for days or weeks following trauma, when the damaged coronary thromboses or ruptures.

If coronary intimal injury is suspected, urgent cardiac catheterization and coronary angiography is indicated. The left anterior descending coronary is most often injured in blunt force trauma, followed by the right coronary artery. The circumflex is rarely injured, and injury to more than one artery has been reported [19].

Management of the coronary injury is dictated by the location and severity of the lesion. Patients with suspected bleeding from an injured coronary should be taken to the operating room for median sternotomy, control of the bleeding site, and coronary bypass to the involved artery. Left main coronary dissections should be treated with coronary bypass or patch angioplasty [20], and percutaneous coronary stenting considered only when associated injuries preclude the use of cardiopulmonary bypass.

In other cases, either percutaneous coronary stenting or coronary bypass can be used to treat the injured coronary artery. If an intimal flap is detected but coronary flow is satisfactory, patients can be managed expectantly, but this option must be carefully weighed against the risk of late thrombosis and the risk of anticoagulation in patients with other severe injuries.

Atrial rupture

Although ventricular rupture may be caused by direct compression of the heart between the sternum and spinal column, tears in the atria are likely caused by abrupt increase in venous pressure by forceful compression of the thorax or abdomen during late systole when the atria are full and the atrioventricular valves are closed. The thin-walled appendages are particularly vulnerable, but tears can also occur at both venocaval-atrial junctions and in the right atrial free wall [21].

Patients with atrial rupture are frequently involved in motor vehicular accidents, and present to the emergency department with hypotension and evidence of tamponade following volume resuscitation [22]. Echocardiography is indispensable in making a timely diagnosis of traumatic rupture of the atrium. These tears can often be repaired without cardiopulmonary bypass by median sternotomy and, in contrast to ventricular rupture, survival is common [23].

Penetrating injuries of the heart

Perhaps the most dramatic of all trauma cases, penetrating injuries of the heart are caused by stab or gunshot wounds, or the rare accidental impalement. Unlike blunt cardiac injuries, which may not be readily apparent in the emergency department, injury of the heart or great vessels should be immediately suspected in any patient with penetrating trauma of the chest. Most patients are unstable in the field and many present to the emergency department receiving cardiopulmonary resuscitation (CPR).

The presentation of patients with penetrating cardiac injuries depends on whether the clinical features of hemorrhage or pericardial tamponade predominate. Knife wounds of the ventricle may seal relatively quickly, and 80% to 90% of patients with stab wounds to the heart present with signs of tamponade [24]. Because the blood in the pericardium clots quickly without defibrination, needle pericardiocentesis may be of little benefit for diagnosis and in reversing tamponade. Mild to moderate amounts of cardiac tamponade can be temporarily overcome by rapid administration of large amounts of fluids while preparations for definitive treatment are undertaken.

In contrast to stab wounds, gunshot wounds of the heart produce large, ragged defects in the cardiac chamber that do not seal readily. Because of the associated defect in the pericardium, tamponade is less likely to occur and the clinical picture is one of severe hemorrhage. Tamponade, when present, is a favorable sign portending a better chance of survival [25].

Approximately 65% of patients with penetrating cardiac injuries have no obtainable blood pressure on arrival in the emergency department [26]. Parameters that are correlate with survival include need for CPR at the scene (negative correlation); the cardiovascular-respiratory score and the Revised Trauma Score itself; systolic blood pressure; and presence of intrapericardial great vessel injury (negative correlation) [27]. In the Los Angeles County–University of Southern California Trauma Center experience, mortality for gunshot wounds involving the heart is more than 85%, and for stab wounds 32% [27].

Management of penetrating injuries of the heart

In any patient with an epigastric or anterior chest wound and hypotension, cardiac injury must be suspected. Fig. 3 presents a reasonable algorithm for management of such patients [24]. If

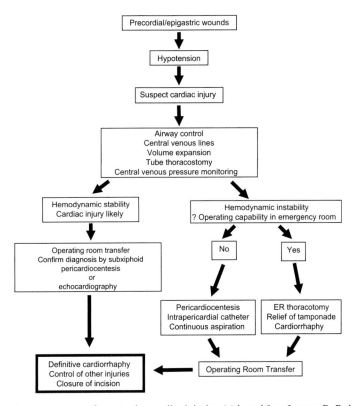

Fig. 3. Algorithm for the management of penetrating cardiac injuries. (*Adapted from* Ivatury R, Rohman M. Penetrating cardiac trauma. In: Turney SZ, Rodriguez A, Cowley RA, editors. Management of cardiothoracic trauma. Baltimore: Williams & Wilkins; 1990. p. 314; with permission.)

the patient is unstable and sternotomy or thoracotomy is not immediately available, subxiphoid pericardiocentesis may be performed as a temporizing measure [25].

Repair of penetrating wounds of the heart can be accomplished through a median sternotomy or left anterior thoracotomy. Sternotomy allows better exposure to right-sided cardiac structures and the right hilum, and permits cannulation for cardiopulmonary bypass if necessary for repair or correction of hypothermia. If there is concern for concomitant injury to posterior structures, however, such as the esophagus or descending aorta or to the left hilum, then left thoracotomy may be preferable.

Following pericardiotomy, lacerations of the atria can be controlled by digital pressure or application of a vascular clamp. A useful technique to control bleeding quickly is insertion of a large Foley catheter directly into the wound followed by inflation of the balloon and gentle traction on the catheter to seal the opening. In the case of right atrial wounds, the Foley can be used

to infuse rapidly intravenous fluids and blood for resuscitation. This method has proved invaluable during emergency room thoracotomies. Injuries to the ventricles are usually repaired with pledgeted sutures, taking care to avoid coronary arteries. In the instance of laceration in the ventricle very near epicardial coronary arteries, placing sutures on either side of the defect and the artery and passing underneath the coronary may allow closure of the injury and avoid compromise of the vessel. Large defects, such as those caused by gunshots, may require a prosthetic patch.

Ventricular septal injury in association with a penetrating cardiac wound may be suspected if the right ventricle appears distended, or if there is a palpable thrill in the right ventricular outflow tract. This injury can be confirmed by oximetry, documenting a step-up in oxygen content between the right atrium and pulmonary artery, or by the use of transesophageal echocardiography. Definitive repair of septal defects should not be undertaken at the time of initial operation, because a number of these defects close spontaneously [28] and because attempts at placing sutures into the ecchymotic and potentially necrotic myocardium can often result in a failed repair.

Although bleeding from small coronary arteries can be controlled by ligation of the injured vessel, there is 40% mortality when this technique is applied to major coronary arteries [29]. In this instance, bleeding can be controlled by placement of intracoronary shunts, such as those used in off-pump coronary bypass procedures. Subsequently, decision can be made to repair the artery by direct suture, vein angioplasty, or ligation and coronary bypass to the distal segment. Late complications of coronary artery injury include coronary-cameral or arterial-venous fistulae and aneurysm formation.

Foreign bodies in the heart

Removal of retained foreign bodies from within the cardiac chambers or embedded in the myocardium was one of the first cardiac operations performed on a routine basis. In 1914, Saurbruch [30] reported a series of 105 patients who had undergone removal of intracardiac foreign bodies. During World War II, Harken [31], the pioneer of intracardiac surgery, successfully removed bullet and shrapnel fragments from in and around the hearts of 100 soldiers without a single operative death.

Generally, removal of foreign bodies from the heart is indicated if there is migration, conduction disturbances, possible gross contamination, or if recurrent pericardial effusions or systemic embolism develop. In the emergency department, fluoroscopy can be used further to evaluate metallic foreign bodies (ie, bullet fragments) that appear on chest radiograph. If the foreign body does not move, then this is suggestive of an intrapericardial location. If the object is located within the myocardium or a chamber of the heart, then sternotomy and cardiopulmonary bypass should used to remove the foreign body to prevent development of complications [32].

Emergency room thoracotomy

Left anterior thoracotomy performed in the emergency department for resuscitation is often perceived as the ultimate heroic effort to save a life. Critics, however, view the procedure as always futile, wasteful, and a needless risk to health care providers in the trauma bay. Although survival following emergency room thoracotomy (ERT) is infrequent, there is a role for this lifesaving technique in select patients. Powell and coworkers [33] reviewed the outcome of ERT in 959 patients treated at Denver Health Medical Center between 1997 and 2003. These authors found that all patients with blunt trauma who required CPR for longer than 5 minutes in the field either died or were neurologically devastated following ERT. In contrast, in patients suffering penetrating trauma and requiring prehospital CPR and subsequent ERT, only 1 of 22 survivors suffered serious neurologic injury. Furthermore, survival for patients presenting to the emergency department with shock and a penetrating cardiac injury was 35% and 15% for all penetrating trauma, as opposed to only 2% for those with blunt trauma and less than 1% for patients with blunt trauma and absent vital signs [34]. ERT is an effective treatment option for patients with penetrating trauma of the chest who present with shock or requiring CPR for less than 15 minutes. ERT is not without significant complications, and is difficult even under optimal conditions. Favorable results can only be expected when ERT is performed by experienced operators. It is essential that trauma teams plan and practice in advance of the moment when emergency thoracotomy might be required.

References

[1] Cicero J, Mattox KL. Epidemiology of chest trauma. Surg Clin North Am 1989;69:15–9.
[2] Sigler LH. Traumatic injury of the heart. Am Heart J 1945;30:459.
[3] Rodriguez A, Turney SZ. Blunt injuries of the heart and pericardium. In: Turney SZ, Rodriguez A, Cowley RA, editors. Management of cardiothoracic trauma. Baltimore (MD): Williams & Wilkins; 1990. p. 261–84.
[4] Fulda G, Brathwaite CE, Rodriguez A, et al. Blunt traumatic rupture of the heart and pericardium: a ten-year experience (1979-1989). J Trauma 1991; 31(2):167–72.
[5] Kerins M, Maguire E, Lacy C. Cardiac luxation: an unusual complication of a log roll. Emerg Med J 2005;22(12):913–5.
[6] Maron BJ, Gohman TE, Kyle SB, et al. Clinical profile and spectrum of commotio cordis. JAMA 2002; 287(9):1142–6.
[7] Wisner DH, Reed WH, Riddick RS. Suspected myocardial contusion: triage and indications for monitoring. Ann Surg 1990;212:82–6.
[8] Tenzer ML. The spectrum of myocardial contusion. J Trauma 1985;25:620–7.

[9] Rajan GP, Zellweger R. Cardiac troponin I as a predictor of arrhythmia and ventricular dysfunction in trauma patients with myocardial contusion. J Trauma 2004;57(4):801–8.

[10] Kaye P, O'Sullivan I. Myocardial contusion: emergency investigation and diagnosis. Emerg Med J 2002;19:8–10.

[11] Weiss RL, Brier JA, O'Connor W, et al. The usefulness of transoesophageal echocardiography in diagnosing cardiac contusion. Chest 1996;109:73–7.

[12] Southam S, Jutila C, Ketai L. Contrast-enhanced cardiac MRI in blunt chest trauma: differentiating cardiac contusion from acute peri-traumatic myocardial infarction. J Thorac Imaging 2006;21(2):176–8.

[13] Pai M. Diagnosis of myocardial contusion after blunt chest trauma using 18F-FDG positron emission tomography. Br J Radiol 2006;79(939):264–5.

[14] Culliford AT. Nonpenetrating cardiac trauma. In: Hood RM, Boyd AD, Culliford AT, editors. Thoracic trauma. Philadelphia: WB Saunders; 1989. p. 211–23.

[15] Banning AP, Pillai R. Non-penetrating cardiac and aortic trauma. Heart 1997;78:226–9.

[16] Kan CD, Yang YJ. Traumatic aortic and mitral valve injury following blunt chest injury with a variable clinical course. Heart 2005;91:568–70.

[17] McDonald ML, Orszulak TA, Bannon MP, et al. Mitral valve injury after blunt chest trauma. Ann Thorac Surg 1996;61(3):1024–9.

[18] Pretre R, Chilcott M. Blunt trauma to the heart and great vessels. N Engl J Med 1997;336:626–32.

[19] Lai C-H, Ma T, Chang T-C, et al. A case of blunt chest trauma induced acute myocardial infarction involving two vessels. Int Heart J 2006;47:639–43.

[20] Harada H, Honma Y, Hachiro Y, et al. Traumatic coronary dissection. Ann Thorac Surg 2002;74(1):236–7.

[21] Hirai S, Hamanaka Y, Mitsui N, et al. Successful emergency repair of blunt right atrial rupture after a traffic accident. Ann Thorac Cardiovasc Surg 2002;8(4):228–30.

[22] Hermans K, Vermeulen J, Meyns B. Isolated rupture of the left atrial appendage after blunt chest trauma. Acta Cardiol 2004;59(6):663–4.

[23] Fang B-R, Kuo L-T, Li C-T, et al. Isolated right atrial tear following blunt chest trauma: report of three cases. Jpn Heart J 2000;41(4):535–40.

[24] Ivatury R, Rohman M. Penetrating cardiac trauma. In: Turney SZ, Rodriguez A, Cowley RA, editors. Management of cardiothoracic trauma. Baltimore (MD): Williams & Wilkins; 1990. p. 311–27.

[25] Moreno C, Moore E, Majure J, et al. Pericardial tamponade: a critical determinant of survival following penetrating cardiac wounds. J Trauma 1986;28:821–5.

[26] Tyburski J, Astra L, Wilson R, et al. Factors affecting prognosis with penetrating wounds of the heart. J Trauma 2000;48(4):587–90.

[27] Asensio J, Murray J, Demtriades D, et al. Penetrating cardiac injuries: a prospective study of variables predicting outcome. J Am Coll Surg 1998;186(1):24–34.

[28] Rosenthal A, Parisi L, Nadas A. Isolated interventricular septal defect due to nonpenetrating cardiac trauma. N Engl J Med 1970;283(7):338–41.

[29] Rea WJ, Sugg WL, Wilson LC, et al. Coronary artery laceration: an analysis of 22 patients. Ann Thorac Surg 1969;7(6):518–28.

[30] Saurbruch F. Die verwendbarkeit des unterdruchverfahrens bei der herz chirurgie. Arch Klin Chirurgie 1907;83:537–42.

[31] Harken DE. Foreign bodies in, and in relation to, the thoracic blood vessels and heart, I: techniques for approaching and removing foreign bodies from chambers of the heart. Surg Gynecol Obstet 1946;83:117–25.

[32] Bland E, Beebe G. Missiles in the heart: a twenty-year follow-up report of World War II cases. N Engl J Med 1996;274(19):1039–46.

[33] Powell D, Moore E, Cothren C, et al. Is emergency department resuscitative thoracotomy futile care for the critically injured patient requiring prehospital cardiopulmonary resuscitation? J Am Coll Surg 2004;199(2):211–5.

[34] Cothren C, Moore E. Emergency department thoracotomy for the critically injured patient: objectives, indications, and outcomes. World J Emerg Surg 2006;24:1–4.

ELSEVIER
SAUNDERS

Thorac Surg Clin 17 (2007) 95–108

THORACIC
SURGERY
CLINICS

Overview of Great Vessel Trauma

William T. Brinkman, MD, Wilson Y. Szeto, MD, Joseph E. Bavaria, MD*

Division of Cardiovascular Surgery, Hospital of the University of Pennsylvania, 3400 Spruce Street, 4 Silverstein, Philadelphia, PA 19104, USA

Injury to the great vessels of the thorax (the aorta and its brachiocephalic branches) can occur following blunt and penetrating trauma. The goal of the surgeon confronted with injuries to these vessels is twofold: the prevention of acute hemorrhage and the prevention of delayed hemorrhage caused by posttraumatic aneurysm or pseudoaneurysm ruptures.

Greater than 90% of injuries to the great vessels of the thorax are caused by penetrating trauma [1]. Gunshots, stab wounds, shrapnel, and even iatrogenic misadventures are frequently reported causes.

The innominate artery, pulmonary veins, vena cavae, and most frequently the thoracic aorta are especially susceptible to blunt injury. Aortic blunt injury usually involves the proximal descending aorta, but other segments, such as the ascending aorta or transverse arch (10%–14%), mid-distal descending aorta (12%), or even multiple sites (13%–18%), have been reported [2,3].

Blunt aortic injury

Incidence

The exact incidence of blunt aortic disruption is not known, but is estimated to be responsible for approximately 8000 deaths per year in the United States [4]. Autopsy series of blunt trauma patients have reported rates of aortic rupture from 12% to 23%. Aortic injury is the second most common cause of death in blunt trauma patients behind brain injury [5]. Vesalius [6], in 1557, was the first to describe a patient death from a ruptured aorta after being thrown from a horse. In large part, however, traumatic blunt aortic injury (BAI) is a disease of modern society. The first successful repair accomplished by Klassen was reported by Passaro and Pace [7] in 1957. Before this report, prominent medical journals advised physicians to avoid surgery for traumatic aortic aneurysms [8]. Parmley and colleagues [9] from the Armed Forces Institute of Pathology in 1958 first emphasized the lethality of the blunt traumatic aortic disruption with a combined autopsy and clinical study. The percentage of death at the accident scene was 85%. Of the patients who made it to the hospital alive most subsequently died from aortic rupture within a few days.

Blunt aortic disruption is primarily caused by motor vehicle accidents and falls. Motor vehicle crashes account for approximately 80% of blunt aortic injuries. Head-on collisions are the most common mechanism, but side and rear impacts were also causes. Patients with BAI tend to be young (mean age, 39 years) [5]. In a review of automobile crashes from the United Kingdom from the 1990s there was 9% survival at the scene with blunt aortic rupture and an overall mortality of 98%. Impact scenarios were variable, but interestingly most common from the side. Interestingly, 81% of fatalities were using either seat belts or air bags at the time of the crash [10]. Falls resulting in aortic injury generally are from 3 m or greater. Substance abuse is common and is present in over 40% of the motor vehicle crashes resulting in aortic disruption. Seatbelt use decreases risk by a factor of four. Ejection from

* Corresponding author.
  E-mail address: joseph.bavaria@uphs.upenn.edu
(J.E. Bavaria).

1547-4127/07/$ - see front matter © 2007 Published by Elsevier Inc.
doi:10.1016/j.thorsurg.2007.02.009

a vehicle doubles the risk of aortic disruption [11,12]. For drivers and front seat passengers, steering wheel deformity is an independent predictor of a serious thoracic injury [13]. Even the use of air bags in automobile crashes has been associated with BAI, in some instances with speeds as low as 10 mph.

Box 1 lists the frequency of associated injuries in patients with BAI in data compiled from the 1970s to the late 1990s. The American Association for the Surgery of Trauma compiled prospective data on 274 cases of BAI from 50 trauma centers throughout the United States and Canada. They reported 50% of patients with BAI have associated brain injury. Other series have reported associated brain injuries as low as 30% [5,14]. Associated chest injuries, pelvic or long bone fractures, and severe abdominal injuries were also frequently reported.

Pathology

Blunt acute aortic disruption

The degree of BAI, first described by Parmley and colleagues [9], is a continuum from subintimal hemorrhage to total aortic disruption. They classified the lesions into six groups: (1) intimal hemorrhage, (2) intimal hemorrhage with laceration, (3) medial laceration, (4) complete laceration of the aorta, (5) false aneurysm formation, and (6) periaortic hemorrhage. Patients who arrive alive to the hospital generally have sustained an incomplete noncircumferential lesion to the media and intima. The tunica adventitia and the mediastinal pleura then prevent free rupture. Unbelievably, there are examples in the literature of patients with complete aortic transections managing to survive long enough to allow intervention [15].

Any part of the aorta, from the aortic root to the iliac bifurcation, can be involved with BAI; however, BAI tends to be confined to a few specific locations. The classic site of BAI is in the descending aorta at the isthmus. BAI may also occur in the ascending aorta proximal to the origin of the brachiocephalic, aortic arch, and distal descending or abdominal aorta. Most patients suffer a single injury, but there are examples of multiple BAIs in a single patient [16]. Autopsy series describe 36% to 54% occur at the aortic isthmus, 8% to 27% at the ascending aorta, 8% to 18% at the arch, and 11% to 21% at the distal descending aorta [3,9,17,18]. Most surgical series demonstrate a much higher percentage of aortic isthmic injuries (80%–100%), and only 3% to 10% in the ascending aorta, arch, or distal descending aorta. This discrepancy of the data suggests that the peri-isthmic aortic adventitia may be more durable than other segments of the aorta, allowing containment of rupture. This assertion is contradicted by tensile tests conducted by Lundevall on aortic wall samples [19].

The several different mechanical forces act in the pathogenesis of BAI. The relative importance of these forces remains a subject of debate.

Stretching. The earliest proposed mechanism of BAI was stretching of the aortic wall. This was supported by tensile test data demonstrating the inherent weakness of the isthmus and the relative immobility of the fixed distal descending aorta relative to the ascending aorta and arch. The isthmus lies at the junction of these two segments.

Box 1. Associated injuries occurring in 274 patients with blunt aortic injury

Closed head: 140 (51)[a]
Multiple rib fractures: 123 (46)
Flail chest: 34 (12)
Pulmonary contusion: 103 (38)
Myocardial contusion: 10 (4)
Diaphragm rupture: 20 (7)
Spleen: 39 (14)
Liver: 61 (22)
Small bowel: 19 (7)
Other abdominal: 38 (14)
Spinal cord: 10 (4)
Pelvis: 84 (31)
Femur: 67 (24)
Tibia: 60 (22)
Upper extremity: 54 (20)
Maxillofacial: 36 (13)
C-spine: 12 (4)
T-spine: 11 (4)
L-spine: 10 (4)
None: —

Numbers in parentheses are percentage of patients with that injury.

[a] Thirty-four (24%) had intracranial hemorrhage.

Data from Fabian T, Richardson J, Croce M. Prospective study of blunt aortic injury: multicenter trial of the American Association for the Surgery of Trauma. J Trauma 1997; 42:374–80.

Against this hypothesis are data showing the aortic wall is capable of sustaining strains of up to 80% before rupture. The area stretched must be very localized to be stretched to the required strain of rupture within the thoracic cage (Fig. 1) [20,21].

Sudden blood pressure elevation. Others have proposed a sudden rise in blood pressure as the cause of BAI. A number of investigators have dismissed this rationalizing that an isotropic cylinder under pressure ruptures longitudinally rather than transversely. Transverse tears (as seen with BAI) occur only if the transverse strength is more than twice the longitudinal strength [15]. Tensile data from Mohan and Melvin [20] on aortic wall samples did demonstrate the transverse to longitudinal strength was almost the required 2:1 ratio. In addition, their test samples consistently failed in a transverse manner. Much of this bench tensile data gives little clinical relevance. Zehnder in 1956 calculated that an intravascular pressure of 2500 mm Hg is necessary to produce rupture of the aorta [22].

Osseous pinch. This novel hypothesis reported by Crass and colleagues [23] proposed that aortic rupture is caused by entrapment of the aorta between the anterior thoracic bony structures and the vertebral column. A similar mechanism was proposed by Symbas [24], who proposed that the aorta was forced onto and stretched over the spine in high-impact injuries.

Water-hammer effect. When flow of a noncompressible fluid is obstructed suddenly, a high pressure reflected wave is generated. If during a vehicle impact the aorta is occluded at the diaphragm suddenly, a reflected wave is generated. The pulse pressure generate by this reflected wave is greatest at the aortic arch because of the curvature reflection and further intensification. This phenomenon has been studied only in simple analytic models [25]. Symbas [21] concluded that torsion stress and stress from the water-hammer effect are most likely responsible for injuries to the ascending aorta and bending and shearing stresses affect the aortic isthmus.

Multivariate hypotheses. More likely is the explanation that a combination of multiple forces including shear, torsion, and stretching combined with hydrostatic forces cause blunt aortic injuries [15].

Chronic traumatic aortic aneurysm

Chronic traumatic aortic aneurysms are rarely found in the clinical setting and natural history data are incomplete. Guidelines for their management are not well delineated in the literature.

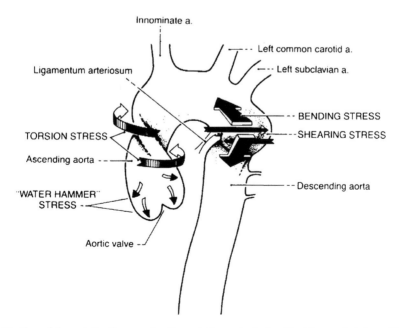

Fig. 1. Demonstration of the putative forces acting through the aorta during blunt traumatic injury. (*From* Symbas P. Cardiothoracic traumas. London: WB Saunders; 1989.)

Most believe that if detected over 2 years from the initial trauma these lesions can be followed for onset of symptoms or radiologic changes. Once the acute period is over their management is similar to a true thoracic aneurysm [26–28]. Rarely, chronic posttraumatic aneurysms have been reported to form fistulas to the pulmonary artery [29] and bronchus [30,31]. Symptomatic compression of mediastinal and hilar structures has also been reported [32].

Open repair of chronic traumatic aneurysms is associated with a mortality rate of 5% to 18% and a morbidity rate of 11% to 50%. More recently, endovascular repair of chronic aortic injuries has been performed using covered stents. Short-term mortality and morbidity is improved with aortic stenting versus open repair, but improvements in long- term outcomes remain to be seen [33]. Mid-term data on the endovascular management of descending aortic aneurysms are promising. Significant reductions in operative mortality have been seen with endovascular approaches to thoracic aneurysms. In addition, reintervention rates and paraplegia rates are similar in open and endovascular cohorts [34].

Clinical presentation

Diagnostic studies

Chest radiograph

Following arrival in the emergency room a supine anteroposterior chest radiograph should be routinely obtained for trauma patients. All emergency room physicians, radiologists, and surgeons should have experience in interpreting supine portable chest radiographs because many patients are clinically unstable or have suspected spinal injuries making upright posteroanterior chest radiographs unsafe. Assessment of a supine chest radiograph can rapidly rule out significant pathology, such as pneumothorax, hemothorax, and fractures. If possible, an upright chest radiograph should be obtained. A normal upright chest radiograph has a negative predictive value of approximately 95% to 98% [35].

When presented with penetrating injuries, marking of entrance and exit sites with radiopaque markers is useful. Radiographic findings suggestive of penetrating great vessel injury include a large hemothorax; foreign bodies or their trajectory close to the great vessels; a confusing trajectory, which may indicate a migrating

endovascular course; or a "missing" missile suggesting embolization [36].

Radiographic findings suggestive of blunt injury to the thoracic aorta include fractures of the sternum, scapula, clavicle, first rib, or multiple left-sided ribs. Indirect mediastinal clues include obliteration of the aortic knob, depression of the left mainstem bronchus, loss of the paravertebral pleural stripe, an apical pleural cap, deviation of a nasogastric tube, and lateral displacement of the trachea at the T-4 level [35]. Pathologic widening of the mediastinum defined as greater than 8 cm at the level of the aortic knob or if the ratio of mediastinal width to chest width exceeds 25% has a reported sensitivity of 81% to 100% and a specificity of 60%. Determination of the presence of mediastinal widening can have a significant inter-reader variability, however, even among experienced radiologists. The radiologist's overall impression regarding the mediastinum and not any one measurement has been found to be a more sensitive predictor of traumatic aortic injury [37].

CT

Contrast-enhanced CT using multidetector-row technology has now replaced angiography as the screening modality for traumatic aortic injury [38]. In the past 5 years there has been a dramatic change in the diagnosis and screening for traumatic aortic injury. Traditional "step and shoot" CT scanners were not deemed acceptable as a screening tool because of slow acquisition, motion artifact, and poor spatial resolution [39]. With the arrival of multidetector-row CT (MDCT), concerns regarding image acquisition time and spatial resolution have been minimized. A MDCT study from the base of the skull through the symphysis pubis can be performed in less than 1 minute.

At many trauma centers, all multitrauma patients receive a MDCT. The protocol used for multisystem evaluation usually includes nonionic contrast at 3 to 4 mL/s for a total volume of 90 to 125 mL. Collimation of 3.2 mm with a pitch of 1.25 is then used to reconstruct images at 1.6-mm intervals. Multiplanar reformulations are then used to evaluate vascular structures including the aorta. Using this protocol at the Ryder Trauma Center over a 4-year period, 48 cases of traumatic aortic injury were identified. All of these 48 cases were diagnosed using direct signs of injury. Direct signs include active extravasation of contrast, pseudoaneurysm formation, intimal flaps, and filling defects. Indirect signs of aortic injury include periaortic hematoma and mediastinal hematoma [40]. Direct signs of aortic injuries have been shown to be more accurate than indirect signs [41]. Traditionally, periaortic hematomas without direct signs on CT were considered suspicious for aortic injury. Aortography was then recommended as a standard of care [42,43]. Since the development of MDCT, the presence of periaortic hematomas in the absence of a direct sign of aortic injury does not necessarily require aortography. This depends, however, on the confidence of the radiologist, the quality of the scanner, and the study [44]. There have been reports of positive aortograms with no direct signs of aortic injury, but all of these cases were performed on older-generation helical scanners, not MDCT [42,43].

The traditional gold standard for the diagnosis of traumatic aortic injury, with sensitivity and specificity approaching 100%, is aortography. Multiple studies using single-slice helical CT for the diagnosis of traumatic aortic injury, however, have shown sensitivities and specificities equal to aortography [45,46]. The ability of MDCT accurately to diagnose aortic injury and injuries to other areas of the body makes it the more useful diagnostic tool in the trauma patient. In addition, MDCT has been proved to be cost effective and is always available. In addition, MDCT can be used for stent graft sizing if an endovascular approach is planned for repair.

Transesophageal echocardiography

Transesophageal echocardiography (TEE) has been demonstrated to be a useful tool for the evaluation of traumatic aortic injury. Multiple authors have demonstrated the ability of TEE to visualize cardiac and vascular structures making it a useful decision-making tool in chest trauma. In addition, TEE can be applied quickly at the bedside or in the emergency room while resuscitation is ongoing. Some authors promote TEE as a first-line test in the initial evaluation of trauma patients involved in high-velocity deceleration injuries, regardless of mediastinal width on chest radiograph.

The accuracy of TEE in the published literature is varied. There are no prospective randomized trials looking at TEE in trauma. In a meta-analysis of studies of TEE in the setting of traumatic aortic injury, however, the sensitivity and specificity of TEE was approximately 97%. When TEE was compared directly with aortography, the sensitivity and specificity of TEE was slightly lower than with aortography (93% versus 95%). The findings of these studies were adversely affected by small enrolment numbers [47–49]. The main findings of this meta-analysis were that TEE has an overall high diagnostic performance for the detection of traumatic aortic injury, and in general application no differences were found in the diagnostic performance of TEE and aortography.

TEE demonstrated better diagnostic performance in patients with small aortic injuries, not requiring surgery. These small aortic lesions can be missed by aortography because they do not cause any change in aortic shape [50]. In addition, these small lesions require careful diagnosis and follow-up because of their unpredictable evolution. Three trials followed patients with minor nonsurgical aortic injuries. In these studies, TEE was consistently positive, whereas in 10 of 12 patients aortography or CT scan was negative. It is unclear whether the use of MDCT would have increased the sensitivity for nonsurgical aortic injuries. In these studies TEE was then used to follow the progressive healing of the nonsurgical aortic lesions. The clinical application of these data is debatable because of the small sample size, inconsistent follow-up, and the unknown sensitivity of TEE for small nonsurgical aortic injury. TEE seems promising, however, for the diagnosis and follow-up of these lesions. Further studies to learn the incidence of nonsurgical BAI, their long-term prognosis, and the role of TEE in their management are necessary [47,49–51].

Unfortunately, TEE requires specific training and expertise and may not be as available as CT or angiography. This can lead to significant time delays in a patient population where rapid decisions are critical. TEE may also be difficult to use in patients with neck injuries or where cervical spine clearance is pending. In addition, TEE does not visualize well the ascending aorta or aortic branches [52,53].

Aortography

Angiography of the aorta is the gold standard for significant BAI, although with the inception of MDCT and TEE this has been questioned. There is a small incidence of false-positive angiograms from known anatomic abnormalities, such as ductus diverticulum and aberrant brachiocephalic arteries. Physicians interpreting angiography should, however, be familiar with these variants [54–56].

Magnetic resonance angiography

Long examination times and limited access have been limitations to the application of MRI in acute aortic pathology. The development of fast MRI techniques (down to a few minutes), however, has now allowed its use even in critically ill patients. The use of MRI in detecting traumatic aortic rupture in comparison with angiography and CT was reported in a series of 24 patients. The diagnostic accuracy was 100% for MRI; 84% for angiography (two false-negatives); and 69% for CT (two false-negatives and three false-positives) [57]. It must be acknowledged that these CT data were not MDCT. MRI is most useful in detecting the hemorrhagic component of a traumatic lesion. An aortic tear limited to the anterior or posterior wall could be visualized and followed if one opted for nonoperative management. Discrimination of the extent of aortic hematoma may be of prognostic significance. MRI currently is not a common test used to evaluate acute injury to the thoracic great vessels. In situations where an aortic injury is being followed nonoperatively, however, MRI can be an excellent tool. This is especially true if there is a contraindication to CT angiography, such as renal insufficiency [58].

Management

Timing of operation

Once the diagnosis of a blunt or penetrating aortic injury is made, immediate repair is recommended. This practice began with the landmark paper from Parmley and colleagues [9]. Most important was their observation that of the 38 patients who made it to the hospital alive, 23 of these died of rupture within 7 days of admission. In their conclusions, they stated that to save life, early diagnosis and immediate surgical intervention was required. In the 1990s, however, Pate and colleagues [59] pointed out that these observations by Parmley and colleagues [9] were in the "presurgical era" and that the injury pattern had since changed [38,59]. Rupture at the aortic isthmus was reported in only 45% of Parmley's cases, whereas recent surgical series are generally over 80% [60–62]. These findings seemed to indicate a change in etiology. Motor vehicle crash is now the most common mechanism for BAI. Moreover, injuries at the aortic isthmus seem to be more stable than other locations of the thoracic aorta [38].

Surgical management in patients with BAI is challenging and associated with operative

mortality rates as high as 30% [5]. Multiple associated severe injuries are common and are most likely the cause of this excess morbidity and mortality. Because of this reality, immediate operative repair may not be possible. The Western Association of Trauma multicenter study group identified age and pre-existing cardiac disease as major contributing factors in operative mortality. They recommended that these patients may benefit from longer preoperative work-up or nonoperative management. They also noted that there was no difference in outcomes if stable patients had operations immediately or if it was delayed longer than 24 hours [63].

Patients who may benefit from initial medical management and delayed surgical repair include those with the following [38,63,64]:

1. Cardiac risk factors: segmental wall motion abnormality on echo, ongoing angina, prior coronary artery bypass graft, and need for inotropic support
2. Head injury: abnormal CT (hemorrhage or edema)
3. Pulmonary injury: pulmonary contusion on imaging combined with Pao_2/Fio_2 <300 mm Hg, or positive end-expiratory pressure requirement of 7.5 cm of H_2o to maintain adequate oxygenation, or inability to tolerate single lung ventilation
4. Coagulopathy: extensive nonsurgical bleeding or INR >1.5 or laboratory evidence of consumption, such as increased fibrin split products or platelets <100,000
5. Severe abdominal solid organ injury and pelvic fractures where the use of heparin may need to be temporarily avoided

Multiple studies have reported the safety of delayed surgical repair of BAI in multitrauma patients by first addressing the life-threatening injury or adopting a nonoperative strategy [38]. Maggisano and colleagues [64] reported a 90% survival rate following delayed aortic repair in 44 patients with severe concomitant injuries or sepsis. Holmes and colleagues [65] in a subgroup analysis of 30 patients with delayed management found 15 patients managed nonoperatively (delayed management was defined as patients who did not undergo operative repair within 24 hours of injury). Three patients exhibited progression of their aortic injury within 5 days of the injury and of these two died. Of the 15 patients managed with a delayed operation, three deaths occurred (one rupture and two intraoperative arrests).

The 15 patients managed without an operation were followed for a mean of 2.5 years. Ten of these 15 patients survived without the need for further surgery; five had complete resolution and five were left with a radiographically stable pseudoaneurysm. The five deaths in the nonoperated patients were all caused by head trauma. They concluded that selected patients with multiple severe associated injuries or high-risk premorbid conditions may undergo delayed aortic repair or nonoperative management. They did, however, mandate serial radiographic examinations during the first week of the hospitalization [65]. Factors that may cause the abandonment of a delayed or nonoperative strategy for BAI include a rapid increase in the size of a mediastinal hematoma or pleural effusion, anuria persisting for more than 6 hours, limb ischemia, or the free leak of contrast media within the thorax. Transient hypotension in association with these signs is an ominous sign and indicates impending rupture [66].

It has become generally recognized that patients admitted with blunt traumatic aortic injuries fall into two distinct categories: stable and unstable. The hemodynamically unstable group has been associated with an all-cause mortality exceeding 90%. The hemodynamically stable group generally is afforded time for work-up and staging of any intervention. The mortality in this group is generally as low as 25% [65]. Fabian and colleagues [67–69] have demonstrated that an aggressive antihypertensive regimen can significantly reduce the rate of rupture in blunt aortic injuries. They recommended maintenance of systolic blood pressure below 100 mmHg or mean arterial pressure less than 80 mmHg and control of heart rate (<100 beats/min) using an intravenous β-blocker, such as esmolol or labetalol. A vasodilator was added if a satisfactory blood pressure was not achieved with β-blockade alone. The combination of a β-blocker with a vasodilator reduces aortic wall shearing force by lowering ventricular ejection dynamic.

Operative management

Besides execution of a technically sound vascular repair, spinal cord protection and distal end organ protection are the predominant concerns during operative repair of a BAI to the aortic isthmus or descending thoracic aorta. The optimal method of spinal cord protection during repair is a source of continued debate in the surgical literature. Traditionally, a "clamp and sew"

approach has been used. It has become clear, however, that cross-clamp times greater than 30 minutes are associated with paraplegia rates of 15% to 30% [5,70].

In general, spinal cord perfusion is dependent on radicular arteries, which arise from the posterior intercostal and lumbar arteries. Collateral blood supply to the cord is supplemented from the left subclavian artery and internal iliac arteries. Because the blood supply to the spinal cord is somewhat variable and the risk of paraplegia is difficult to predict in any given patient, a spinal protective strategy is important in all patients. In the lower thorax and upper abdomen the anterior spinal artery is less well developed. This increases the reliance on adjacent intercostal and lumbar arteries. In 25% of patients, the artery of Adamkiewicz (which arises anywhere from T8–L4) is essential for lower thoracic spinal cord perfusion because of discontinuity of the anterior spinal artery [71,72].

Important etiologic factors of postoperative paraplegia are the duration of cross-clamp, the level and length of aorta excluded by the cross-clamp, the perfusion pressure of the aorta distal to the cross-clamp, increased cerebrospinal fluid pressure, total body and spinal cord temperature, systemic arterial hypotension, and the number of intercostal arteries ligated during surgery. Of note, patients with traumatic aortic injury do not have a well-developed collateral circulation to the spinal cord in contrast to patients with coarctation and chronic aneurysmal disease of the aorta [38,59]. Increasing spinal cord blood flow with shunts, oxygenated bypass circuits, cerebrospinal fluid drainage, intrathecal administration of vasodilators, and reattachment of intercostals arteries have been used with varied success in the prevention of spinal cord ischemia. Pharmacologic measures have included hypothermia, anesthetic agents, calcium channel blockers, free radical scavengers, and immune system modulation [73].

Von Oppell and colleagues [74] in a meta-analysis of spinal cord protection during aortic surgery in the absence of collateral circulation noted the risk of paraplegia increased progressively as the cross-clamp time lengthened if simple aortic cross-clamping was used. They noted a cutoff time of 30 minutes of cross-clamp where the rate of paraplegia began to increase markedly if no method of distal perfusion was used. The rates of paraplegia in their meta-analysis were 19% with simple cross-clamp application; 8.2% if passive distal perfusion was used; and 2.3% if active augmentation of distal aortic perfusion was used ($P < .00001$ versus simple cross-clamp application or passive shunts). Mortality was higher in polytraumatized patients when they were perfused distally with methods requiring full systemic heparinization (18.2%), however, compared with methods not requiring full heparinization (11.9%; $P < .01$) [74].

Management of spinal and lower body circulation

Passive and active augmentation of distal aortic circulation

The use of passive augmentation of distal circulation to decrease postoperative paraplegia was first reported by Gott in 1972 [75]. Following this, Molina and colleagues [76] published experimental data indicating that the passive flow provided by the Gott shunt was inadequate consistently to prevent paraplegia. The length of the tube and inner diameter were constraints to adequate flow. To address these limits imposed by the laws of fluid dynamics, Oliver and colleagues [77] used heparin-bonded tubing between the left atrium and the femoral artery and a centrifugal pump to achieve active augmentation of distal perfusion. In their first nine cases reported there were no instances of paraplegia. The benefits of active distal perfusion during aortic cross-clamp in reducing spinal cord injury have been supported by multiple surgical series [5,78–80]. Forbes and colleagues [79] in a review of 30 patients who underwent repair of descending aortic transections reported no neurologic deficits in the 21 patients who had distal perfusion, whereas four of the nine patients who underwent clamp and sew had new neurologic deficits. Read and colleagues [80] subsequently reported a retrospective series of 16 consecutive patients with descending aortic disruptions repaired with left heart bypass and a centrifugal pump. They demonstrated an 88% operative survival and no cases of paraplegia. Fabian and colleagues [5] reported prospective data on 207 cases of stable BAI undergoing repair. Twelve of the 73 patients treated with clamp and sew developed paraplegia, whereas only 6 of the 134 patients treated with left heart bypass had postoperative paraplegia ($P < .004$) They concluded that distal aortic perfusion significantly lowered paraplegia rates compared with a clamp and sew approach.

Most series have failed to demonstrate a clear benefit of active distal perfusion, however, because of poor statistical power [60]. Some authors still advocate the clamp and sew technique. Sweeney and colleagues [81] reported a series of 71 patients undergoing repair of traumatic aortic injuries with an average cross-clamp time of 24 minutes, overall mortality of 12%, and a paraplegia rate of 1.5%. In experienced hands good results can be obtained with a simple clamp and sew technique. In actual surgical practice it is impossible to predict whether a repair can be performed in less than 30 minutes. Only 33% of the repairs in the prospective analysis of North American repairs of BAI reported by Fabian and colleagues [5] in 1997 were under 30 minutes.

Spinal cord injury following repair of blunt injury of the descending aorta and isthmus generally occurs either during operative repair or during the postoperative period. Interruption of blood flow with aortic cross-clamping is believed to be the causative event. Hypertension proximal to the aortic cross-clamp occurs if no measures are taken to unload the left ventricle. This hypertension can result in the production of increased spinal fluid and may decrease spinal cord perfusion [82]. Delayed paraplegia can manifest, however, up to 21 days following repair. This delayed response is believed to be from intraoperative hypotension followed by reperfusion injury to the cord. The duration of cross-clamp has also been shown to be related to the duration of ischemia [82].

Some surgeons have advocated left atrial–femoral bypass (LA-FA or left heart bypass) versus femoral vein–femoral artery partial cardiopulmonary from bypass (FA-FV) techniques as better in the prevention of postoperative paraplegia. Believed advantages of LA-FA are left ventricular unloading, distal perfusion, and the need for minimal or no heparinization in LA-FA circuits. Unloading of the left heart can be especially important in the setting of a concomitant myocardial contusion. If 1 L/min flow and a distal aortic pressure of 50 mm Hg are maintained, systemic heparin is not required in most LA-FA circuits. There have been reports of posterior cerebral infarctions associated with the LA-FA circuits used without heparin where the cross-clamp times exceeded 30 minutes [83]. Because of this, most surgeons use 10,000 units of heparin if clamp times are expected to exceed 30 minutes [84]. The two main disadvantages of LA-FA bypass are occasional injury to the left atrial appendage or pulmonary veins and occasional inadequate pump flows. FA-FV bypass is the use of partial cardiopulmonary bypass using a pump and oxygenator with full heparinization. FA-FV bypass minimizes the occurrence of hypoxia, which can be critical in the setting of one lung ventilation, pulmonary contusion, and insufficiency. In addition FA-FV bypass provides excellent distal perfusion while decreasing preload to the heart. The main disadvantage of FA-FV bypass is the need for full heparinization. A retrospective analysis by Weiman and colleagues [84] in 2006 showed a higher paraplegia rate in patients being repaired with LA-FA bypass versus FA-FV bypass. This difference, although not significant, occurred even with decreased cross-clamp times in the LA-FA group. Full heparinization in multitrauma patients should be used cautiously and has been associated with increased mortality in some series.

Location of the aortic cross-clamp is also an important factor in preserving spinal cord perfusion. Commonly, the proximal aortic clamp site in an open aortic transection repair is between the left common carotid and the left subclavian artery. With application of a clamp proximal to the left subclavian, important collaterals to the spinal cord (eg, the internal mammary artery) are occluded. Active augmentation of distal perfusion can minimize spinal cord ischemia while a beveled anastomosis incorporating the left subclavian artery is fashioned.

Endovascular stent graft repair

Even with recent advances in surgical and anesthetic techniques, the open repair of traumatic aortic injuries is still associated with significant morbidity and mortality. Because of this the use of thoracic endovascular stent grafts (TEVAR) for repair of BAI is currently being investigated [85]. Endovascular stent grafts have been used for the definitive treatment of infrarenal aortic aneurysms since 1991 with excellent results. Stimulated by this success, endovascular technology is now being applied to diseases of the thoracic aorta [86–92].

Multiple series with limited patient numbers and limited follow-up indicate that TEVAR is a viable alternative to open repair for traumatic aortic injuries. Perioperative mortality and paraplegia rates seem to compare favorably with traditional open repair. These results are apparent despite increased intercostal artery occlusion and frequent coverage of the left subclavian artery compared with open repair. The reason for this is unclear, but it may be because mean arterial

pressures can be run higher after stent repair versus open repair.

Leurs and colleagues [93], in an analysis of the EUROSTAR database, reported on 50 patients treated with traumatic aortic transections (Fig. 2). They reported an operative mortality of 6% and a paraplegia rate of 6%. Reed and coworkers [94] recently reviewed their experience with traumatic transections over a 5-year period from 2000 to 2005. A total of 51 patients presented with the diagnosis of traumatic transection. Twenty-seven (52%) patients died before intervention. Of the remaining 24 patients, 9 patients underwent emergent conventional open repair. Thirteen patients underwent delayed TEVAR, with the mean duration from diagnosis to treatment of 6 days. Technical success with complete exclusion of the transection was achieved in all 13 patients. Thirty-day mortality was 23% (N = 3). Tehrani and coworkers [95] reported their experience of 30 patients with traumatic aortic

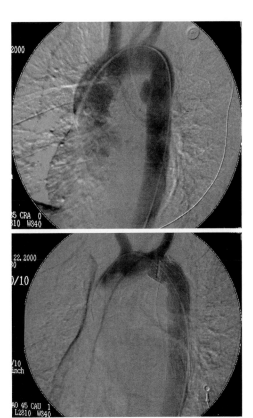

Fig. 2. Traumatic aortic transection before and following endovascular stent graft repair. The stent proximal margin is distal to the left subclavian artery.

transection and severe concomitant nonaortic injuries treated with TEVAR. Technical success was 100% with angiographic evidence of complete exclusion of the disruption. There were two perioperative deaths and no incidence of paraplegia. With a mean follow-up of 11.6 months, there was no evidence of endoleak, stent migration, or late pseudoaneurysm formation [95]. Other smaller series have demonstrated similar findings, with a mean follow-up period up to 21 months [89,96–98]. Perioperative mortality rates ranged from 0% to 11%, with no incidence of paraplegia. All endovascular stent graft deployment was performed using none or low-dose heparin. Stroke was rare, with one series reporting one patient suffering a cerebrovascular accident [89,92,96,98].

In emergent and urgent cases, the anatomy of the vertebral, carotid, and vertebrobasilar system usually is not known. Coverage of the left subclavian artery in the acute situation is generally well tolerated. Mild ischemic symptoms may be noted postrepair. In these patients, a subsequent left subclavian to left common carotid bypass can be performed in a later procedure [89]. Arm ischemia following repair of acute aortic transections is relatively rare and generally well tolerated. The main question, however, is the chance for increased ischemic damage to the posterior cerebral circulation with vertebral artery occlusion.

The most useful applicability of endovascular technology seems to be for patients with severe nonaortic blunt injuries who would otherwise be denied surgical repair of the aortic injury. TEVAR in this group of severely injured patients may not significantly improve overall survival, however, with these patients eventually succumbing to their associated nonaortic traumatic injuries. More evidence and long-term follow-up are needed before definitive conclusions can be made. Early and midterm results are promising with an endovascular approach. It must be noted, however, that these repairs must be followed with serial imaging unlike traditional open repairs. Long-term follow-up data are needed to define better the role of TEVAR in acute aortic transections. It seems apparent that even if long-term success is not equivalent to open repair, the ability to convert an emergent or urgent intervention to a later elective repair is a benefit to the multitrauma patient.

The current generation of thoracic stent grafts was designed for aneurysmal disease processes. Because aortic size in an acute transection is usually normal, currently available thoracic stent grafts are occasionally too large for endovascular repair. In these situations, extension cuffs used from abdominal aneurysm supplies can be used.

Nonisthmic aortic and arterial lacerations

Rupture of the ascending and transverse aorta is uncommon, but the exact incidence is unknown because of the lethality of these injuries. A widened mediastinum and cardiac tamponade are frequently associated with ascending aortic ruptures. Repair of ascending aortic injuries requires full heparinization by a median sternotomy. The management of the aortic tear may be primary or with interposition graft. Special attention to the status of the aortic valve should be maintained. Injuries to the aortic arch may require the use of hypothermic circulatory arrest and associated antegrade and retrograde cerebral perfusion techniques. Survival primarily depends on the severity of associated injuries [99,100].

Innominate artery injuries generally can be repaired by a median sternotomy with a right cervical extension when necessary. Blunt injury typically involves the base of the innominate artery. This is most expeditiously repaired with bypass to the distal innominate from the ascending aorta followed by oversew of the innominate base. Division of the innominate vein is occasionally required for exposure. Shunts or cardiopulmonary bypass should not be needed. Avoidance of the injured area until completion of the bypass leads to a technically easier repair [101].

Subclavian vascular injuries require preoperative imaging for appropriate incision planning. Injuries to the right subclavian are best addressed by a median sternotomy with a right cervical extension. Proximal control of left-sided subclavian injuries can be obtained by a left anterior thoracotomy. A separate supraclavicular incision can be used for distal control. These two incisions can be connected with a sternotomy to facilitate exposure (the "book" thoracotomy). This incision should be used sparingly because of a reported incidence of postoperative causalgia neurologic symptoms [102,103].

The surgical approach to injuries of the left carotid artery mirrors that of the innominate with the use of a sternotomy with a left cervical extension if needed. With injuries of the left carotid origin bypass graft repair is generally preferred over end-to-end reanastomosis [36].

Endovascular approaches to innominate, intrathoracic carotid, and subclavian arterial injuries have also been described [104–108]. The long-term results of this approach are not known, but it can be an attractive option in the multi-trauma patient who is not a good candidate for a traditional open repair.

Summary

Traumatic injury to the aorta and the brachio-cephalic branches are potentially lethal injuries. Specialized preoperative imaging and medical management can lead to better outcomes in this group of patients. In addition, improved surgical techniques for spinal cord protection have led to decreased morbidity in surgical candidates. TE-VAR remains a promising technique; however, long-term data currently are not available.

References

[1] Mattox K, Feliciano D, Beal A. Five thousand seven hundred and sixty cardiovascular injuries in 4459 patients: epidemiologic evolution 1958–1988. Ann Surg 1989;209:698–705.

[2] Williams JS, Graff JA, Uku JM, et al. Aortic injury in vehicular trauma. Ann Thorac Surg 1994;57(3): 726–30.

[3] Feczko J, Lynch L, Pless J, et al. An autopsy case review of 142 nonpenetrating (blunt) injuries of the aorta. J Trauma 1992;33:846–9.

[4] Nagy K, Fabian T, Rodman G, et al. Guidelines for the diagnosis and management of blunt aortic injury. In: Bromberg W, editor. Trauma practice guidelines. East Northport (NY): The Eastern Association for the Surgery of Trauma; 2000.

[5] Fabian T, Richardson J, Croce M. Prospective study of blunt aortic injury: multicenter trial of the American Association for the Surgery of Trauma. J Trauma 1997;42(3):374–80.

[6] Vesalius A. Sepulchretaum sive Anataomia Practica ex Cad a veribus Morbo, T. Beonetus, Editor. 1700 [in Italian].

[7] Passaro E, Pace W. Traumatic rupture of the aorta. Surgery 1957;46:787–91.

[8] Steinberg I. Chronic traumatic aneurysm of the thoracic aorta: report of five cases, with a plea for conservative treatment. N Engl J Med 1957;257: 913–8.

[9] Parmley L, TW M, Manion T. Nonpenetrating traumatic injury of the aorta. Circulation 1958; XVII:1086–101.

[10] Richens D, Kotidis K, Neale M, et al. Rupture of the aorta following road traffic accidents in the United Kingdom 1992–1999: the results of the co-operative crash injury study. Eur J Cardiothorac Surg 2003;23(2):143–8.

[11] Dischinger P, Cowley R, Shankar B. The incidence of ruptured aorta among vehicle fatalities. Proc Assoc Adv Automot Med Conf 1988;32:15.

[12] Greendyke RM, Greendyke RM. Traumatic rupture of aorta: special reference to automobile accidents. JAMA 1966;195(7):527–30.

[13] Newgard CD, Lewis RJ, Kraus JF, et al. Steering wheel deformity and serious thoracic or abdominal injury among drivers and passengers involved in motor vehicle crashes [see comment]. Ann Emerg Med 2005;45(1):43–50.

[14] Hilgenberg A, Logan D, Akins C, et al. Blunt injuries of the thoracic aorta. Ann Thorac Surg 1992;53:233–8.

[15] Richens D, Field M, Neale M, et al. The mechanism of injury in blunt traumatic rupture of the aorta. Eur J Cardiothorac Surg 2002;21(2):288–93.

[16] Brundage S, Harruff R, Jurkovich G, et al. The epidemiology of thoracic aortic injuries in pedestrians. J Trauma 1998;45:1010–4.

[17] Arajarvi E, Santavirta S, Tolonen J. Aortic ruptures in seat belt wearers. J Thorac Cardiovasc Surg 1989;98:355–61.

[18] Rabinsky I, Sidhu G, Wagner R. Mid-descending aortic traumatic aneurysms. Ann Thorac Surg 1990;50:155–60.

[19] Lundevall J. Traumatic rupture of the aorta, with special reference to road accidents. Acta Pathol Microbiol Scand 1964;62:29–33.

[20] Mohan D, Melvin J. Failure properties of passive human aortic tissue. J Biomech 1982;15(11): 887–902.

[21] Symbas P. Cardiothoracic traumas. London: W.B Saunders; 1989.

[22] Kirklin J, Barrett-Boyes B. Cardiac surgery. London: Churchill Livingstone; 1993.

[23] Crass J, Cohen A, Motta A, et al. A proposed new mechanism of traumatic aortic rupture: the osseous pinch. Radiology 1990;176:645–9.

[24] Symbas P. Fundamentals of clinical cardiology: great vessel injury. Am Heart J 1977;93:518–22.

[25] Ray G, Liu Y, N D. Wall stress in curved aorta in blunt-chest trauma. 28th Annual Conference on Engineering in Medicine and Biology. Alliance for Engineering in Medicine and Biology. September 20–24, 1975.

[26] Kondo N, Koyama M, Wakayama F, et al. Surgical repair for chronic traumatic thoracic aneurysm after 12-year follow-up. Jpn J Thorac Cardiovasc Surg 2004;52(12):586–8.

[27] Bacharach JM, Garrett LM, Rooke TW, et al. Chronic traumatic thoracic aneurysm: report of two cases with the question of timing for surgical intervention. J Vasc Surg 1993;17(4):780–3.

[28] Katsumata T, Shinfield A, Westaby S, et al. Operation for chronic traumatic aortic aneurysm: when and how? Ann Thorac Surg 1998;66(3):774–8.

[29] Hirose H, Svensson LG. Chronic posttraumatic aneurysm of descending aorta with fistulous

communication into pulmonary artery. J Vasc Surg 2004;40(3):564–6.

[30] Pantaleo P, Prothero T, Banning AP, et al. Aorto-bronchial fistula resulting from an accidental fall one year earlier. Int J Cardiol 1999;68(2): 239–40.

[31] Fernandez Gonzalez AL, Montero JA, Luna D, et al. Aortobronchial fistula secondary to chronic post-traumatic thoracic aneurysm. Tex Heart Inst J 1996;23(2):174–7.

[32] Baba M, Yashamita A, Sugimoto S, et al. [A case of a chronic traumatic thoracic aneurysm with compression of left main bronchus at the isthmus]. Kyobu Geka 1998;51(10):860–3 [in Japanese].

[33] Gawenda M, Landwehr P, Brunkwall J, et al. Stent-graft replacement of chronic traumatic aneurysm of the thoracic aorta after blunt chest trauma. J Cardiovasc Surg 2002;43(5):705–9.

[34] Stone D, Brewster D, Kwolek C, et al. Stent-graft versus open-surgical repair of the thoracic aorta: mid-term results. J Vasc Surg 2006;44:1188–97.

[35] Mirvis S, Bidwell J, Buddenmeyer E, et al. Value of chest radiography in excluding traumatic aortic rupture. Radiology 1987;163:487–93.

[36] Mattox K, Wall M, LeMaire S. Injury to the great thoracic vessels. In: Mattox K, Feliciano D, Moore K, editors. Trauma. New York: McGraw-Hill; 2000.

[37] Ho R, Blackmore C, Bloch R. Can we rely on mediastinal widening on chest radiography to identify subjects with aortic injury? Emerg Radiol 2002;9: 183–7.

[38] Nzewi O, Slight R, Zamvar V. Management of blunt thoracic aortic injury. Eur J Vasc Endovasc Surg 2006;31:18–27.

[39] Miller F, Richardson J, Thomas H. Role of CT in diagnosis of major arterial injury after blunt thoracic trauma. Surgery 1989;106:596–602.

[40] Rivas LA, Munera F, Fishman JE. Multidetector-row computerized tomography of aortic injury. Semin Roentgenol 2006;41(3):226–36.

[41] Fishman J, Nunez D, Kane A. Direct versus indirect signs of traumatic aortic injury revealed by helical CT: performance characteristics and interobserver agreement. AJR Am J Roentgenol 1999; 172(4):1027–31.

[42] Mirvis S, Shanmugathan K, Miller B. Traumatic aortic injury: diagnosis with contrast enhanced CT - five-year experience at a major trauma center. Radiology 1996;200:413–22.

[43] Dyer D, Moore E, Mestek M. Can chest CT be used to exclude aortic injury? Radiology 1999;213: 195–202.

[44] Mirvis S, Shanmugathan K. Imaging in trauma and critical care. Philadelphia: Saunders; 2003.

[45] Dyer D, Moore E, Ilke D. Thoracic aortic injury: how predictive is mechanism and is chest tomography a reliable screening tool? J Trauma 2000;48(4): 673–82.

[46] Scaglione M, Pinto A, Pinto F. Role of contrast-enhanced helical CT in the evaluation of acute thoracic aortic injuries after blunt chest trauma. Eur Radiol 2001;11(12):2444–8.

[47] Minard G, Schurr M, Croce M. A prospective analysis of transesophageal echocardiography in the diagnosis of aortic disruption in trauma patients without enlarged mediastinum. J Trauma 1996; 40:225–30.

[48] Chirillo F, Totis O, Cavarzerani A. Usefulness of transthoracic and transesophageal echocardiography in recognition and management of cardiovascular injuries after blunt trauma. Heart 1996;75: 301–6.

[49] Cinnella G, Dambrosio M, Brienza N, et al. Transesophageal echocardiography for diagnosis of traumatic aortic injury: an appraisal of the evidence. J Trauma 2004;57:1246–55.

[50] Goarin J, Cluzel P, Gosgnach M, et al. Evaluation of transesophageal echocardiography for the diagnosis of traumatic aortic injury. Anesthesiology 2000;93:1373–7.

[51] Vignon P, Boncoeur MP, Francoi B, et al. Comparison of multiplane transesophageal echocardiography and contrast-enhanced helical CT in the diagnosis of blunt traumatic cardiovascular injuries. Anesthesiology 2001;94:615–22.

[52] Mollod M, Felner J. Transesophageal echocardiography in the evaluation of cardiothoracic trauma. Am Heart J 1996;132:841–9.

[53] Ahrar K, Smith D, Bansal R. Angiography in blunt thoracic injury. J Trauma 1997;42:665–9.

[54] Morse S, Glickman M, Greenwood L. Traumatic aortic rupture: false-positive aortographic diagnosis due to atypical ductus diverticulum. Am J Roentgenol 1988;150:793–6.

[55] Sturm J, Hankins D, Young G. Thoracic aortography following blunt chest trauma. Am J Emerg Med 1990;8:92–6.

[56] Pozzato C, Gedriga E, Donatelli F, et al. Acute posttraumatic rupture of the thoracic aorta: the role of angiography in a 7-year review. Cardiovasc Intervent Radiol 1991;14:338–41.

[57] Fattori R, Celletti F, Bertacinni P. Delayed surgery of traumatic aortic rupture: role of magnetic resonance imaging. Circulation 1996;94: 2865–70.

[58] Gavelli G, Canini R, Bertaccini G, et al. Traumatic injuries: imaging of thoracic injuries. Eur Radiol 2002;12:1273–94.

[59] Pate J, Fabian T, Walker W. Acute traumatic rupture of the aortic isthmus: repair with cardiopulmonary bypass. Ann Thorac Surg 1995;59:90–9.

[60] Tatou E, Steinmetz E, Jazayeri S, et al. Surgical outcome of traumatic rupture of the thoracic aorta. Ann Thorac Surg 200;69:70–73.

[61] Gammie J, Shah A, Hattler B, et al. Traumatic aortic rupture: diagnosis and management. Ann Thorac Surg 1998;66:1295–300.

[62] Galli R, Pacini D, Bartolomeo R, et al. Surgical indications and timing of repair of traumatic ruptures of the thoracic aorta. Ann Thorac Surg 1998;65: 461–4.

[63] Camp P, Shackford S. The Western Trauma Association Multicenter Group. Outcome after blunt traumatic aortic laceration: identification of a high-risk cohort. J Trauma 1997;43:413–22.

[64] Maggisano R, Nathens A, Alexandrova N, et al. Traumatic rupture of the thoracic aorta: should one always operate immediately? Ann Vasc Surg 1995;9:44–52.

[65] Holmes J, Bloch R, Hall A, et al. Natural history of traumatic rupture of the thoracic aorta managed nonoperatively: a longitudinal analysis. Ann Thorac Surg 2002;73:1149–54.

[66] Simon B, Leslie C. Factors predicting early hospital death in blunt thoracic aortic injury. J Trauma 2001;51:906–11.

[67] Pate J, Gavant M, Weiman D, et al. Traumatic rupture of the aortic isthmus: program of selective management. World J Surg 1999;23:59–63.

[68] Pate J, Fabian T, Walker W. Traumatic rupture of the aortic isthmus: an emergency? World J Surg 1995;19:119–26.

[69] Fabian T, Devis K, Gavant M, et al. Prospective study of blunt aortic injury: helical CT is diagnostic and antihypertensive therapy reduces rupture. Ann Surg 1998;227:666–77.

[70] Von Oppell U, Dunne T, DeGroot M, et al. Traumatic aortic rupture: twenty-year meta analysis of mortality and risk of paraplegia. Ann Thorac Surg 1994;58:585–93.

[71] Adams H, Von Geertruyden H. Neurologic complications of aortic surgery. Ann Surg 1956;144: 574.

[72] Gharagozloo F, Larson J, Dausmann MJ, et al. Spinal cord protection during surgical procedures on the descending thoracic and thoracoabdominal aorta: review of current techniques. Chest 1996; 109(3):799–809.

[73] Mauney MC, Blackbourne LH, Langenburg SE, et al. Prevention of spinal cord injury after repair of the thoracic or thoracoabdominal aorta. Ann Thorac Surg 1995;59(1):245–52.

[74] von Oppell U, Dunne TDG, KM, et al. Spinal cord protection in the absence of collateral circulation: a meta-analysis of mortality and paraplegia. J Cardiac Surg 1994;9(6):685–91.

[75] Gott V. Heparinized shunts for thoracic vascular operation. Ann Thorac Surg 1972;14:219–20.

[76] Molina J, Cogordan J, Einzig S, et al. Adequacy of ascending aortic descending aortic shunt during cross-clamping of the thoracic aorta from prevention of spinal cord injury. J Thorac Cardiovasc Surg 1985;90:126–36.

[77] Oliver H, Maher T, Liebler G, et al. Use of the Biomedicus centrifugal pump in traumatic tear of the thoracic aorta. Ann Thorac Surg 1984;38:586–91.

[78] Walls JT, Curtis JJ, McKenney-Knox CA, et al. Centrifugal pump support for distal aortic perfusion during repair of traumatic thoracic aortic injury. Artif Organs 2002;26(11):991–3.

[79] Forbes AD, Ashbaugh DG. Mechanical circulatory support during repair of thoracic aortic injuries improves morbidity and prevents spinal cord injury. Arch Surg 1994;129(5):494–7 [discussion: 497–8].

[80] Read RA, Moore EE, Moore FA, et al. Partial left heart bypass for thoracic aorta repair: survival without paraplegia. Arch Surg 1993;128(7):746–50 [discussion: 750–2].

[81] Sweeney M, Young D, Frazier O, et al. Traumatic aortic transections: eight year experience with the "clamp-sew" technique. Ann Thorac Surg 1997; 64:384–7.

[82] Moore WM Jr, Hollier LH. The influence of severity of spinal cord ischemia in the etiology of delayed-onset paraplegia. Ann Surg 1991;213(5): 427–31 [discussion: 431–2].

[83] Duke B, Moore E, Moore F, et al. Posterior circulation cerebral infarcts associated with repair of thoracic aortic disruptions using partial left heart bypass. J Trauma 1997;42:1135–9.

[84] Weiman D, Garbuz A, Gursky A, et al. Comparison of spinal cord protection utilizing left atrial-femoral with femoral-femoral bypass in patients with traumatic rupture of the aortic isthmus. World J Surg 2006;30:1638–41.

[85] Schumacher H, Bockler D, von Tengg-Kobligk H, et al. Acute traumatic aortic tear: open versus stent-graft repair. Seminars in Vascular Surgery 2006; 19(1):48–59.

[86] Appoo JJ, Moser WG, Fairman RM, et al. Thoracic aortic stent grafting: improving results with newer generation investigational devices. J Thorac Cardiovasc Surg 2006;131(5):1087–94.

[87] Brooks M, Loftus I, Morgan R, et al. The Valiant thoracic endograft. J Cardiovasc Surg (Torino) 2006;47(3):269–78.

[88] Fattori R, Nienaber CA, Rousseau H, et al. Results of endovascular repair of the thoracic aorta with the Talent Thoracic stent graft: the Talent Thoracic Retrospective Registry. J Thorac Cardiovasc Surg 2006;132(2):332–9.

[89] Kaya A, Heijman RH, Overtoom TT, et al. Thoracic stent grafting for acute aortic pathology. Ann Thorac Surg 2006;82(2):560–5.

[90] Khamaisi M, Anner H, Marincheva G, et al. Stent graft in treatment of penetrating thoracic aortic ulcer. J Am Soc Echocardiogr 2006;19(6):835, e4–6.

[91] Onitsuka S, Tananka A, Akashi H, et al. Initial and midterm results for repair of aortic diseases with handmade stent grafts. Circ J 2006;70(6):726–32.

[92] Wheatley GH III, Gurbuz AT, Rodriguez-Lopez JA, et al. Midterm outcome in 158 consecutive Gore TAG thoracic endoprostheses: single center

experience. Ann Thorac Surg 2006;81(5):1570–7 [discussion: 1577].

[93] Leurs LJ, Bell R, Degrieck Y, et al. Endovascular treatment of thoracic aortic diseases: combined experience from the EUROSTAR and United Kingdom Thoracic Endograft registries. J Vasc Surg 2004;40(4):670–9 [discussion: 679–80].

[94] Reed AB, Thompson JK, Crafton CJ, et al. Timing of endovascular repair of blunt traumatic thoracic aortic transections. J Vasc Surg 2006;43(4):684–8.

[95] Tehrani HY, Peterson BG, Katariya K, et al. Endovascular repair of thoracic aortic tears. Ann Thorac Surg 2006;82(3):873–7 [discussion: 877–8].

[96] Orford VP, Atkinson NR, Thomson K, et al. Blunt traumatic aortic transection: the endovascular experience. Ann Thorac Surg 2003;75(1):106–11 [discussion: 111–2].

[97] Peterson BG, Longo GM, Matsumura JS, et al. Endovascular repair of thoracic aortic pathology with custom-made devices. Surgery 2005;138(4):598–605 [discussion: 605].

[98] Marty-Ane CH, Berthet JP, Branchereau P, et al. Endovascular repair for acute traumatic rupture of the thoracic aorta. Ann Thorac Surg 2003;75(6):1803–7.

[99] Symbas P, Horsley W, Symbas P. Rupture of the ascending aorta caused by blunt trauma. Ann Thorac Surg 1998;66:113–7.

[100] Serna D, Miller J, Chen E. Aortic reconstruction after complex injury of the mid-transverse arch. Ann Thorac Surg 2006;81:1112–4.

[101] Graham J, Feliciano D, Mattox K. Innominate vascular injury. J Trauma 1982;22:647.

[102] Graham J, Feliciano D, Mattox K. Management of subclavian vascular injuries. J Trauma 1980;20:537.

[103] Mattox K. Approaches to trauma involving the major vessels of the thorax. Surg Clin North Am 1989;69:77.

[104] Szeto W, Fairman R, Acker M, et al. Emergency endovascular deployment of stent graft in the ascending aorta for contained rupture of innominate artery pseudoaneurysm in a pediatric patient. Ann Thorac Surg 2006;81:1872–5.

[105] Chandler T, Fishwick G, Bell P. Endovascular repair of a traumatic innominate artery aneurysm. Eur J Vasc Endovasc Surg 1999;18:80–2.

[106] Axisa B, Loftus I, Fishwick G, et al. Endovascular repair of an innominate artery false aneurysm following blunt trauma. J Endovasc Ther 2000;7:245–50.

[107] Joo J, Ahn J, Chung Y, et al. Therapeutic endovascular treatments for traumatic carotid artery injuries. J Trauma 2005;58:1159–66.

[108] Castelli P, Caronno P, Piffaretti G, et al. Endovascular repair of traumatic injuries of the subclavian and axillary arteries. Injury 2005;36(6):778–82.

ELSEVIER
SAUNDERS

Thorac Surg Clin 17 (2007) 109–128

THORACIC
SURGERY
CLINICS

The Endovascular Approach to Acute Aortic Trauma

Riyad Karmy-Jones, MD[a],*, Stephen Nicholls, MD[a],
Thomas G. Gleason, MD[b]

[a]Heart and Vascular Center, Divisions of Cardiac, Vascular and Thoracic Surgery,
Southwest Washington Medical Center, SWMC Physicians Pavilion, Suite 300,
200 N.E. Mother Joseph Place, Vancouver, WA 98664, USA
[b]Center for Thoracic Aortic Disease, UPMC Heart, Lung, and Esophageal Surgery Institute,
Cardiothoracic Surgery, University of Pittsburgh School of Medicine, 120 Lyton Avenue,
Suite m060, Pittsburgh, PA 15213, USA

The treatment of aortic rupture has significantly evolved since Parmley's and coworkers [1] landmark 1958 paper. Based on this report, there was a period between 1960 and the mid-1980s when the standard of care required immediate angiography followed by immediate operative repair, regardless of associated injuries, because the assumption was that these lesions were almost uniformly fatal if not repaired immediately. This fatalistic assessment has undergone significant change. It is now recognized that there are three broad categories of patients: (1) those who die at the scene (70%–80% of the whole); (2) those who present unstable or become unstable (2%–5% of the whole, with a mortality of 90%–98%); and (3) those who are hemodynamically stable and are diagnosed 4 to 18 hours after injury (15%–25% of the whole, with a mortality of 25%, largely caused by associated injuries) [2]. Early institution of β-blockade and pressure control in stable patients to prevent rupture during the initial period, and in selected cases to allow optimization of associated injuries to reduce operative risk, has provided an increased margin of safety [3,4]. Certain minimal injuries can reliably be expected to heal as long as the patient's condition allows tight blood pressure control [3,5,6]. There have also been modifications in operative technique, including an increased use of

mechanical circulatory support and modifications in devices that permit much lower doses of heparin. These measures reduce (but do not eliminate) the risks of paralysis, end-organ failure, and acute cardiac collapse, and have been associated with improved outcomes [7–9].

The incidence of traumatic aortic disruption varies from center to center. Looking at all trauma-related mortality, blunt aortic rupture may be second only to head injury as the primary cause of death. Despite this, accepting that there are approximately 8000 cases per annum in the United States, and given that as many as 85% of victims die at the scene, then only 1000 to 1500 cases per annum survive to be treated. In one of the largest contemporary series, 274 patients were admitted to 50 institutions over 2.5 years. If these cases were distributed evenly, the average institution would have seen only 2.2 cases per annum [10]. In practice, some centers may manage 8 to 15 cases per annum, whereas most may encounter one to two at most. It does seem that the use of seat belts, air bags, and chest protectors has resulted in an increased number of patients surviving motor vehicle and cycle crashes with both fewer associated injuries and smaller aortic defects [11,12].

Amidst this era of improved operative outcomes and medical management, endovascular stent grafts have become a possible third option. In North America, the concept of thoracic endografting, as an extension of abdominal endograft technology, was greatly stimulated by the Stanford group [13,14]. Their initial primary interest, and

* Corresponding author.
E-mail address: karmy@myuw.net
(R. Karmy-Jones).

indeed the bulk of the literature since, was with atherosclerotic aneurysms. It is now known that endografting is an attractive option that can avoid the morbidity of a thoracotomy in patients with multiple injuries, and that it seems to reduce the risk of paralysis [15–17]. Some centers have seen dramatic improvements in outcome using the endovascular approach [18–20]. As with all invasive procedures, there are specific complications and anatomic considerations that need to be incorporated into the planning of endovascular treatments of traumatic thoracic injuries. This article compares outcomes of endovascular approaches with open repair; reviews pertinent anatomy, imaging techniques, and approaches; and discusses complications and their management.

Outcomes of endovascular stents used in the trauma setting

A number of series have been published that support the notion that endovascular stents, in the setting of traumatic aortic disruption, have low mortality (predominantly related to associated injuries) and essentially no risk of postprocedure paralysis. When reviewing these data, it is important to consider the span of time in which the experience was accrued (because stent technology has changed significantly over the past few years); recognize the difference between the acute (whether defined as within 24 hours of injury or longer period) versus chronic; and consider what were the indications for stent grafting and contraindications to open repair. Those series published between 2002 and 2006 (11 reports), comprising 167 patients, the youngest being 16 years of age, have been selected [6,16,17,21–29]. These series ranged from 5 to 30 cases, over time periods ranging from 1 to 7 years. Average follow-up among the 10 series with at least 1 year follow-up was 24 months. Virtually all stents were industry made, although they varied between dedicated thoracic stents and a variety of cuff extenders. There were seven (4%) deaths, two of which were procedure related (one collapse and rupture, one stroke). Type I endoleak occurred in eight instances (4.7%), two healing spontaneously, six requiring further stenting or balloon dilation. There were two iliac ruptures reported, and three (1.7%) cases of acute stent collapse requiring operative intervention. There were two cases of nonfatal stroke and one of brachial occlusion requiring thrombectomy. There were no reports of postprocedure paralysis. In the series of five cases presented by Thompson and coworkers [23], the mean blood loss was 200 mL, there were no complications, and at average follow-up of 20 months all patients were doing well. Peterson and associates [26] reported 11 cases managed acutely with cuff extenders, seven of which were able to be placed completely percutaneous. There were no complications acutely or at average follow-up of 21 months. Dunham and colleagues [28] noted that in patients with isolated chest injuries the length of stay in the ICU and total hospitalization was as low as 1 and 7 days, respectively. These experiences, in combination with an overall major nonfatal complication rate (excluding endoleak) of 4.3% and mortality of 3.6%, justifies the excitement that endovascular approaches have provoked in the management of traumatic aortic rupture. In addition, endografts may also be used not as a definitive repair, but in complicated cases as a bridge to definitive treatment in selected patients who are not suitable candidates for either operative repair or medical management [21].

Comparison between endovascular and open repair

It is inherently difficult retrospectively to compare two techniques that are not necessarily applied to the same patient population with respect to risk assessment, operative experience, and institutional biases. Each center has sufficiently different patient populations and management strategies to make it difficult to make broad generalizations based on an individual study. Again, recognizing that this is not a complete review of all available works, the authors reviewed five papers, published between 2004 and 2006, that specifically compared outcomes within their respective institutions between the two approaches [6,11,17,22,30]. A total of 108 patients underwent open repair. There were 15 deaths (14%) and 4 (4%) cases of new postoperative paralysis. Ninety-three patients underwent endovascular repair, with nine (9%) mortality and no paralysis or paraplegia. Only one death was procedure related among the stent graft group (acute stent collapse).

Rousseau and colleagues [6] compared the outcomes of 35 patients repaired operatively with 29 managed with endografts, and a further 6 managed medically. Among the open-repair group, 28 underwent immediate repair with mortality of 21% and paralysis of 7% compared with no mortality or paralysis among patients operated on in a delayed fashion. Among the 29 patients managed endovascularly, the only morbidity was a ruptured iliac artery, with successful repair without complications at a mean follow-up of 46 months. The six patients with minimal aortic injuries managed medically all survived without complications.

Andrassy and associates [22] reviewed their experience involving 46 patients over 14 years. There was essentially no difference in survival between the two approaches if managed acutely (13.3% endovascular versus 18.8% open) or more chronically (0% for both). The endovascular group experienced a 12.5% conversion to open repair rate, but there were no instances of neurologic deficit. Open repair was associated with two cases of paraplegia and three minor neurologic events, for an overall neurologic complication rate of 22.7%.

Lebl and colleagues [17] compared outcomes between 10 patients who underwent open repair, 8 managed medically, and 7 managed endovascularly. Of note, whereas the team managing these patients did not change, the paper did cover a paradigm shift from open to endovascular repair as the primary modality at that institution. The patients were relatively well matched, however, with no significant differences in Injury Severity Score or age between the groups, although the operative group tended to be younger (39 ± 5 years open versus 59 ± 8 years). There were no appreciable differences in mortality (20% open, 25% medical, 14% stent-graft) and no reports of neurologic complications, but patients undergoing endovascular stenting did have shorter length of stay compared with those undergoing open repair (28 versus 46 days, $P < .5$).

These small comparisons demonstrate that, when feasible, in at least the population over 18 to 20 years, endovascular repair seems to be associated with a markedly lower paralysis rate than open repair, that length of stay may be reduced compared with open repair, but that acute outcome is probably more related to overall injury severity than approach.

Endovascular repair versus medical management

Institution of strict anti-impulse therapy should occur once the diagnosis of aortic rupture is suspected [6,31]. The ideal blood pressure depends on the patient's age and presenting blood pressure. Until recently, the goal was a systolic blood pressure of less than 120 mm Hg or mean arterial pressure less than 60 to 70. More recently, it has been argued that a blood pressure of "less than what the patient was admitted with" may be more appropriate [2,32]. When strict blood pressure control is implemented, in stable patients, the risk of rupture in the first week may be as low as 5% or less [2]. Some series have noted improved outcomes with both delayed open and endovascular repair, but this may reflect some selection bias [6]. Reasons for delaying operative intervention include severe head injury, blunt cardiac injury, solid organ injury, or acute lung injury [8,33]. In these instances, the authors have favored serial surveillance imaging (usually with CT angiography) every 48 hours for 7 to 10 days, to detect any change in the size or character of the lesion [3]. Although the natural history of residual psuedoaneurysms seems to follow those of nontraumatic atherosclerotic aneurysms, these lesions should not, especially in young patients, be considered completely benign, and the authors favor early intervention as soon as medically stable.

Tight medical control of blood pressure may not be possible in every case. Many patients require other interventions, and monitoring and controlling blood pressure during these can be difficult. There are some hazards including renal and splanchnic insufficiency, and secondary brain injury especially in the setting of increased cranial pressure [34]. Although there is some controversy as to the value of driving up cerebral perfusion pressure, or assuming that an increased pressure translates to improved cerebral perfusion, there is general consensus that high pressure is associated with a lower risk of secondary brain injury [35–38]. Closed head injury associated with evidence of increased intracranial pressure (by CT or intracranial pressure monitoring) may actually mandate operative or endovascular repair. One significant advantage of endovascular repair over both operative and nonoperative management is that after the stent is placed, in most cases it is possible to allow blood pressure to normalize, or even increase without the risk of bleeding or rupture. The risk of rupture, even with serial CT angiography and tight hemodynamic control, is not zero. Endovascular stents may be ideally used exactly in these patients who cannot undergo open operative repair because of significant comorbidities.

The extent of injury may also impact the choice between medical and endovascular management. Minor aortic injuries, involving only small intimal defects, often heal without residual defects [5,39].

Even small lesions can go on to rupture, however, if blood pressure is not controlled [3]. If blood pressure can be reasonably controlled, and there are no contraindications to medical management, small intimal defects should be managed medically with close follow-up. Even small pseudoanerysms, in some cases, have healed [3]. Although endovascular management seems to be an ideal solution in patients with significant co-morbidities, and who are judged to be at too high risk for prolonged medical management, it is not clear that this approach is better than medical management in patients with minimal injuries. One simple guideline is that if the lesion is minimal enough such that one would not consider open operative repair, then one should not rush either to endovascular repair.

Endografts currently available

The characteristics of an endograft designed for the thoracic aorta, as opposed to the abdominal aorta, include a long enough delivery system to reach the distal arch from the femoral artery, and flexibility to accommodate the curvature of the arch. There are variations between different types of graft in how they deploy, whether or not proximal or distal components are bare, whether or not they contain hooks, and how they are actually released from the constraining devices. In general, there has been a shift away from deploying devices in aortic trauma (and type B dissection), which rely on uncovered proximal landing zones because of concerns of aortic perforation [40]. An important consideration is that the average young trauma patient has an aortic diameter in the 20-mm range, which is too small for these devices, which were designed for older, atherosclerotic aortas [41]. Secondly, the use of endografts in the acute trauma setting is considered to be off-label by the Food and Drug Administration outside of trials. Currently, there is only one device approved by the Food and Drug Administration for use in the thoracic aorta, and then only for atherosclerotic aneurysms. There are ongoing high-risk trials to determine and prove the use of stent grafts in the trauma setting, and endografts used currently in Europe, Canada, and Australia are under active evaluation in the United States and will soon be available outside of trials. The Gore Thoracic Aortic Graft (W.L. Gore and Associates, Flagstaff, Arizona) is constructed from expanded polytetra fluoro ethylene, wrapped

in self-expanding nitinol stents that have a suture-less attachment. There is a radiopaque band at each end, with 0.5-cm proximal and distal extension flares covered to assist in wall apposition (Fig. 1). These flares can be placed partially across an orifice without occluding the orifice. The device is introduced through a 30-cm sheath, the outer diameter varying depending on the diameter of the graft. The delivery catheter is fairly flexible and 100 cm in length (Table 1). The device is released by pulling a rip cord that unlaces the constraining system with rapid (less than a second) release starting in the center. This central deployment prevents a windsock effect, and there is rarely any need critically to lower blood pressure during deployment to beyond normal ranges to prevent distal migration. When advancing the catheter, there can be built-up tension, and so the device should be advanced just beyond the proposed landing zone and then brought back into the proper alignment just before deployment. One characteristic of the Thoracic Aortic Graft device is that it rarely if ever jumps forward. Rather, it may drop a millimeter or two back (distally). In appropriately sized patients, the Thoracic Aortic Graft offers an exceptionally good approach because of its flexibility and rapid deployment characteristics [11,42].

Two other companies, Cook and Medtronic, have also been developing and refining endografts for use in the thoracic aorta, and the early iterations, like the Gore, have proved very useful in trauma patients in Europe, Canada, and Australia [24,25,28,30,43,44].

The Cook-Zenith TX2 (Cook, Bloomington, Indiana) is made of woven polyester fabric over

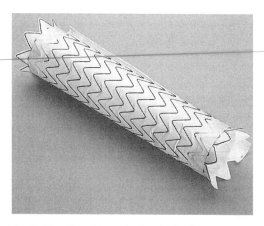

Fig. 1. The Gore Thoracic Aortic Graft (*Courtesy of* W.L. Gore and Associates, Flagstaff, Arizona).

Table 1
Characteristics of the Thoracic Aortic Graft

Stent Diameter (mm)	Length (cm)	Landing zone inner diameter (mm)	Introducer size (Fr)	Access vessel diameter (mm)
26	10	23	20	7.6
28	10	24–26	20	7.6
	15			
31	10	26–29	22	8.3
	15			
	20			
34	10	29–32	22	8.3
	15			
	20			
37	10	32–34	24	9.1
	15			
	20			
40	10	34–37	24	9.1
	15			
	20			

stainless steel Z-stents. The TX2 has a proximal form, which has no bare stents but does have 5-mm long barbs. The distal component does have a bare metal distal segment (Fig. 2). The proximal device can be uniform or tapered. The diameters range from 28 to 42 mm (in 2-mm increments) and the lengths vary from 120 to 216 mm (Table 2). The tapered form narrows at the third Z-stent and the distal diameter is 4 mm less than the proximal (see Table 2). The sheaths are precurved, and 75 cm long. A 20-Fr catheter sheath (OD 23 Fr) is used for 28- to 34-mm stents, and a 22-Fr catheter sheath (OD 25 Fr) for 38- to 42-mm endografts. Although it is rare to need it in the trauma setting, the TX2 is designed with a distal component, to allow modification of the distal portion of the graft to fit the anatomic requirements of the distal landing zone. This portion has an uncovered bare area. The device is unsheathed, but three trigger wires continue to constrain the device, reducing any windsock effect, and allowing final careful positioning before complete release.

The Medtronic Talent Thoracic graft has recently been released in Europe in a modified form, the Valiant (Medtronic, Santa Rosa, California). The Valiant differs in that although it is still made of a low-profile polyester monofilament material, the nitinol stents are on the outside, and with two proximal configurations, one covered and the other with 12-mm flexible bare stents to allow adaptation to the aortic curvature and greater fixation. In addition, there has been improved conformability of the distal end, which may be covered or have a bare extension (FreeFlo)

(Fig. 3, Table 3). Medtronic tends to recommend the FreeFlo model over the covered proximal stent because the experience, at least with non-traumatic aortic pathology, is that the increased

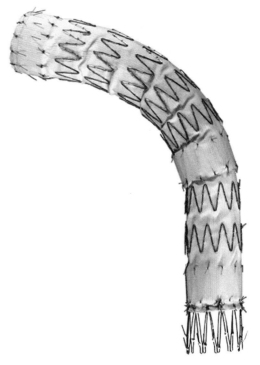

Fig. 2. The Cook-Zenith TX2 Graft with proximal and distal components. (*Courtesy of* Cook, Bloomington, Indiana).

Table 2
Characteristics of the Cook-Zenith TX2 proximal component

Nontapered

Diameter (mm)	Length (mm)	Introducer Sheath (Fr-ID)
28	120	20
	140	
	200	
30	120	20
	140	
	200	
32	120	20
	140	
	200	
34	127	20
	152	
	202	
36	127	22
	152	
	202	
38	127	22
	152	
	202	
40	108	22
	135	
	162	
	216	
42	108	22
	135	
	162	
	216	

Tapered

Proximal Diameter (mm)	Distal Diameter (mm)	Length (mm)	Introducer Sheath (Fr-ID)
32	28	160	20
		200	
34	30	157	20
		197	
36	32	157	22
		197	
38	34	152	22
		202	
40	36	158	22
		208	
42	38	158	22
		208	

flexibility allows the uncovered portion to conform well to the aorta, leading to better fixation. Like the Cook-TX2, the Valiant comes in both a proximal and distal component, although with short lesions, the proximal component alone is often sufficient. Both come in straight or tapered versions. The delivery system involves an unsheathing maneuver. The device allows retraction

and repositioning to permit exact placement. The Talent does come in a slightly smaller model than the Valiant (22 mm), which may be useful in aortas with diameters of 18 to 19 mm.

Because of the size constraints in the typical trauma patient, and because the arch is often acutely angled, some groups have used abdominal aortic cuff extenders rather than dedicated

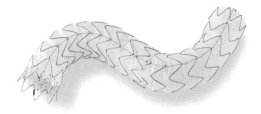

Fig. 3. The Valiant Thoracic Graft with proximal and distal components together. (*Courtesy of* Medtronic, Santa Rosa, California.)

thoracic aortic stent grafts [26,29,45]. These are not only smaller, but may actually fit the aortic configuration of transected aortas better, albeit at the expense of needing multiple grafts, of an increased risk of type III endoleak, and of having to use the shorter delivery system that is designed for the infrarenal aorta [46]. The AneuRx (Medtronic, Santa Rosa, California) cuff extenders range from 20- to 28-mm diameter; are 4 cm long; and are delivered through a 21-Fr catheter, which is 59 cm long. The Gore-Excluder aortic cuffs (W.L. Gore and Associates, Flagstaff, Arizona) are 3.3 cm long; have diameters of 23, 26, and 28.5 mm; and can be delivered by an 18-(for the 23-mm device) or 20-Fr catheter sheath, which is 61 cm long. On occasion, a contralateral limb or iliac extender from an abdominal aortic set may fit the specific anatomic requirements.

Preoperative and procedural imaging

At the outset, it is important to recall that plain chest radiograph is the primary screening tool for patients who have sustained a severe-deceleration injury, but it is generally accepted that between 2% and 7% of patients with a traumatic rupture have a normal chest radiograph initially. Some centers have found higher false-negative rates and emphasize the importance of mechanism in predicting the need for CT angiography [47–49]. If a patient is unstable with pelvic injuries, angiography is performed. The site of pelvic bleeding is controlled first, and then arch angiography is performed [11,50]. In most cases, CT angiography should be performed, and it has at least the sensitivity and specificity of angiography [31,51,52]. CT angiography usually provides all the data necessary to make the diagnosis and treatment plan. Should the diagnosis be made and a pelvic view not taken, then a noncontrast CT of the pelvis should be obtained to evaluate the adequacy of the femoral and iliac arteries for access. Currently, if hematoma is noted around the great vessels, their origin, or the arch, but no definite injury is seen, the authors recommend angiography to exclude associated great vessel injury [53,54]. Transesophageal echocardiography has also been used to make the diagnosis, although its sensitivity of 57% to 63% and specificity of 84% to 91% is less than that reported with CT angiography

Table 3
Characteristics of the Talent-Valiant Graft

Proximal end	Distal end	Proximal diameter (mm)	Covered length (cm)	Catheter size (Fr)
Straight section				
FreeFlo	Closed Web	24,26,28,30,32	100,150	22
FreeFlo	Closed Web	30,32	200	22
FreeFlo	Closed Web	34,36,38,40	100,150,200	24
FreeFlo	Closed Web	42,44,46	100,150,200	25
Closed Web	Closed Web	24,26,28,30,32	100,150	22
Closed Web	Closed Web	30,32	200	22
Closed Web	Closed Web	34,36,38,40	100,150,200	24
Closed Web	Closed Web	42,44,46	100,150,200	25
Closed Web	Bare Spring	24,26,28,30,32	100	22
Closed Web	Bare Spring	34,36,38,40	100	24
Closed Web	Bare Spring	42,44,46	100	25
Tapered section (distal diameter is 4 mm less than proximal)				
Closed Web	Closed Web	28,30,32	150	22
Closed Web	Closed Web	34,36,38,40	150	24
Closed Web	Closed Web	42,44,46	150	25

[55]. Transesophageal echocardiography can be performed during emergent laparotomy, can evaluate cardiac function, and can be used to confirm small defects and differentiate between pre-existing ulcerated plaques and a true aortic injury [55–58]. Intravascular ultrasound has been used in a similar fashion [59,60]. Both transesophageal echocardiography and intravascular ultrasound can also be used to measure aortic diameters and location of the great vessels, site of injury, and so forth [57,59,61]. The authors' bias has been to use intravascular ultrasound in the setting of chronic aneurysm arising from a traumatic injury, if only because in the emergent setting it adds another step.

Most traumatic injuries are located within 2 cm of the origin of the left subclavian artery, and are in proximity to the arch. To visualize the anatomy properly, the most open view of the arch should be obtained. In younger patients, usually a left anterior oblique view at the 60- to 90-degree range is required. The optimal angle can be estimated from the CT angiography (Fig. 4). During angiography, using a multimarker pigtail catheter, one can be confident that the optimal view has been obtained when

the marks are equidistant throughout the image. This facilitates the most accurate positioning of the proximal graft and determines the length of coverage needed.

Accessing either brachial artery for angiograms or marking with a wire has been advocated by some groups [21]. This can augment precise localization of the graft relative to the origin of the left subclavian. Alternatively, in patients with severe acute arch angulation, placing a stiff wire from the right side may permit straightening during deployment [21]. The authors have not used the right brachial approach in the trauma setting, because of concerns of dissection or stroke.

Patient positioning is critical. The arms can obscure visualization of the relevant anatomy. Options include abducting them above the head or placing a roll under the left side to gain some 10 degrees. If it is anticipated that brachial catheterization is needed, the arm should be prepared out. Before preparing and draping the patient, fluoroscopy in key anticipated views should be quickly done to make sure that there are no leads in the way, and that the arch can be easily seen without obstruction.

Anatomic considerations

Anatomic considerations are listed in Table 4. The initial factor to determine is the diameter of the proximal and distal landing zones. Measurements are taken from inner wall to inner wall. The diameter can be difficult to assess in the distal arch, but one method is to measure the transverse diameter at its widest point. In younger adults the aorta is relatively uniform through the arch. Three-dimensional reconstruction and measurements of the descending aorta just at the level of the main pulmonary artery can help confirm estimations of the proximal landing zone diameter. The stent graft diameter should be approximately 10% to 14% larger than the landing zone diameters.

Because most transections occur in proximity to the left subclavian, the next decision is whether or not to cover the subclavian origin. Deploying the graft within the distal curve (gray zone) of the arch may result in partial occlusion of the aorta, increase the risk of stent migration or collapse, and result in an endoleak (see Fig. 4; Figs. 5 and 6). The origin of the left subclavian artery can be marked and both the "drop down" distance measured based on the number of cuts of the

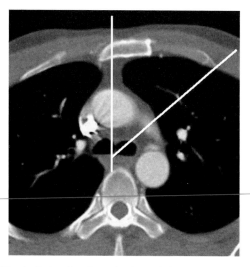

Fig. 4. Estimating the optimal angulation during angiogram. A line is drawn in the anteroposterior direction, and a second through the mid portion of the arch. In this case, a 45-degree left anterior oblique projection should give a good view of the arch. The lesion's location may require a 90-degree oblique view to see it clearly, however, and the left arm may be in the way unless the patient's left side is bumped up or the arms are retracted over their head.

Table 4
Anatomic considerations

Anatomic features to consider	Implications
Diameter of proximal and distal landing zones	Determines size of endograft that can or should be used
Distance from lesion to origin of left subclavian artery	Will obtaining an adequate landing zone require coverage of the left subclavian artery?
Distance from lesion to origin of left common carotid artery	If required, is there room to land distal to the origin of the left common carotid artery? Will there be room, if needed, to clamp distal to the origin or will circulatory arrest be needed if subsequent operative repair is needed?
Degree of curvature across the proximal landing zone	Is there a high likelihood that to avoid malposition along the inner curvature that the graft will have to placed more proximally?
Quality of the aorta	Is there significant thrombus or calcification that poses a risk of stroke or type I endoleak?
Quality of access vessels	Is the diameter sufficient to permit the required sheath? Are there more proximal calcifications or tortuosity that might prevent safe passage of the sheath?
Distance from proposed access vessel to the lesion	Does the system being used have sufficient length to reach the proposed site?
Length of the injury	If using cuffs, how many may be required to ensure fixation?
Vascular anomalies	Anomalous origin of left vertebral artery? Patent LIMA graft? Aberrant origin of right subclavian artery?

CT and the transverse measurement should be estimated. Ideally, at least 2 cm of proximal and distal landing zone is recommended, but in some younger patients, with otherwise normal aortas, 1 cm has proved acceptable.

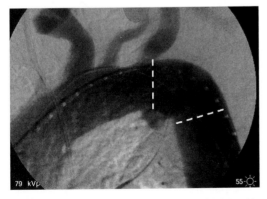

Fig. 5. The "gray zone" or "no man's land." In this case, there is a 90-degree angulation. If the endograft lands between the lines, the proximal end may traverse across the aortic lumen, increasing the risk for collapse, migration, or endoleak. To get an adequate landing zone not only to cover the lesion but also to sit properly in the arch, the left subclavian artery may need to be covered.

The proximal aortic landing zone and arch needs to be reviewed to assess for the presence of significant thrombus or calcification. Focal areas of calcification can result in elevating a lip of endograft, resulting in increased risk of proximal endoleak. Significant thrombus increases the risk of stroke and distal embolization.

The length of the aorta that needs to be covered is based on a minimum of a 2-cm landing zone. If using cuff extenders, usually three are required to provide stability [29,46].

Having chosen the optimal size and type of endograft, the next consideration is the length of the delivery device. Commercial thoracic endograft delivery systems have sufficient length to reach the entire thoracic aorta from the femorals, but cuff extenders have delivery systems of only 61 cm, which may not reach from the groin to the arch. Additionally, the quality and diameter of the proposed access arteries need to be evaluated. The diameter, angulation, and degree of calcification should be determined. Calcifications are better seen with noncontrast images. A noncalcified vessel may tolerate a slightly oversized sheath, but a severely calcified vessel may not accept a sheath that is predicted to fit based on size criteria alone.

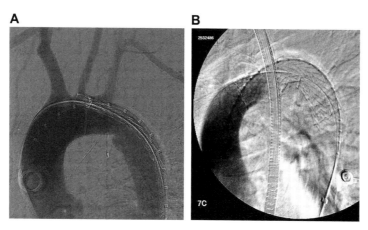

Fig. 6. (*A*) As the endograft is advanced, in this case it seeks the outer curve of the aorta, and one can anticipate that the proximal end will be generally well apposed to both the inner and outer aortic walls. (*B*) This postdeployment image shows the benefit of pushing on the stiff wire to help the endograft lie against the outer curvature. The multiholed pigtail is being pushed too so that it curves against the greater curvature. The stiff wire over which the device was advanced was pushed in a similar fashion but postdeployment has fallen back into its normal line. Had the endograft not been encouraged to form along the outer curvature, the graft might have deployed in a more straight line, resulting in loss of apposition along the inner curvature.

Borsa and colleagues [41] reviewed the anatomic features of 50 trauma patients with documented traumatic aortic rupture who underwent angiography. The average age was 37 years. The mean distance between the superior aspect of the injury and the origin of the left subclavian artery was 5.8 mm along the inner curve and 14.9 mm along the outer curve. The mean diameter adjacent to the injury was 19.2 mm. The mean degree of curvature from the left subclavian artery and the inferior aspect of the injury was 54 degrees. The mean length of the injury was 17 mm along the inner wall and 26 mm along the outer wall. In addition, the injury involved one quarter of the circumference in 44%, one half in 16%, three quarters in 18%, and the complete circumference in 22%. Finally, 28% had a bovine arch and 10% had aberrant origin of the left vertebral artery from the arch proximal to the left subclavian artery. The implications of this study are that given currently available technology, at least 50% of patients require coverage of the left subclavian artery to obtain even minimally acceptable landing zone, and at least 50% or more of patients are not candidates for the Thoracic Aortic Graft but require smaller-diameter devices.

Coverage of the left subclavian artery origin with subclavian to carotid bypass or transposition raises the question of arm ischemia, vertebral-basilar insufficiency, or type II endoleak. Critical arm ischemia is rare, affecting less than 2% of

patients, and if it occurs can be managed electively in most cases [16,42,44,62,63]. Type II endoleak arising by back flow into the pseudoaneurysm is also uncommon because most tears arise from the inner curve. Should type II endoleak occur, or if there is concern before the procedure, the left brachial artery can be accessed and once the graft is deployed, the subclavian can be coiled or closed with a peripheral closure device [64]. Vertebral steal phenomenon can also be addressed electively [65]. Patients with patent left internal mammary grafts should undergo carotid-subclavian bypass before left subclavian coverage [42,65].

Impeding the flow to the left vertebral may pose a risk of posterior cerebellar circulatory insufficiency or stroke. In the authors' experience this has never happened in the younger population, but there is concern in older patients with diffuse vascular disease. Assessing cerebral circulation is clearly difficult under emergent conditions. Anatomic assessments can be made by CT angiography or MR angiography of the head and neck, or cerebral angiography either before or at the time of placement. The authors have found transcranial Doppler to be a useful adjunct. If the basilar artery and the posterior communicating artery can be seen, then flow from both vertebral arteries, the basilar arteries, and posterior communicating arteries can be measured while temporally occluding the origin of the left subclavian artery with an occlusion balloon. Demonstrating intact vertebral-basilar flow on left subclavian occlusion precludes the need for prophylactic subclavian bypass, or transposition is not needed [66].

Carotid-subclavian bypass is generally well tolerated, but some investigators have noted an increased stroke risk when this is performed in patients with atherosclerotic aneurismal disease [65,67]. This may be related to the increased degree of calcification in this older population, and may not apply to the younger trauma patient. The authors' bias is to assess cerebral circulation, but if the case is emergent, and there is no gross evidence of diffuse calcification, the subclavian is covered if needed without waiting for further imaging, and if subsequent vertebral-basilar or arm ischemia results, it is treated electively.

If the proximal landing zone is believed to encroach on the origin of the left subclavian, but complete coverage is not required, it is possible to access the left brachial artery and leave a wire in the arch, which allows precise placement of the device and can permit stenting of the subclavian origin if narrowing occurs [25].

Femoral, iliac, and aortic access

Access vessel choice depends on size of sheath required for the chosen endograft, length of delivery system, quality and diameter of the arteries, and clinical setting. Most trauma patients have healthy vasculature, and slight mismatch can be tolerated between sheath size and femoral diameter as long as there is no tugging and the sheath advances easily under fluoroscopy. If there is any concern, a contralateral sheath should be placed so that balloon occlusion can be used in the event of an iliac rupture during sheath removal. A variety of devices have been used for percutaneous closures with good results [29]. These devices are designed to place intra-arterial sutures that are then tied down at the end of the case [68]. The most common device used, the Perclose (Perclose/Abbott Laboratories, Redwood, California), places two sutures at right angles to each other. They are placed over a wire at the start of the case, and in general most clinicians prefer to tie them down over a glide wire at the end so that if there is a failure of closure a sheath can be reintroduced and a cutdown performed. There is an approximately 10% to 20% failure rate with these devices, which are designed generally for sheaths smaller than those used during endografting procedures. The authors have found that

accessing the femoral artery under ultrasound guidance permits one to be sure they are indeed in the common femoral artery, are anterior, and to avoid areas of calcification or thrombus. When using sheaths required for dedicated thoracic stent grafts, the authors use two placed at 90 degrees to each other. Complications include infection, arterial thrombosis, and pseudoaneurysm, and collectively occur at a rate of about 5%. There are no significant differences between the devices [69–73]. Percutaneous approaches can be performed as quickly as a cutdown if the operators have experience, but in emergency situations or if there are any concerns regarding the quality of the femoral artery (calcification, size, and so forth), then a cutdown is safer. The groin incision can be oblique, at or above the groin skin crease, or longitudinal. If there are extensive calcifications, such endografts as the Thoracic Aortic Graft have been advanced without using the sheath, but this is not recommended because the graft can catch on an edge and deploy prematurely or be damaged. When withdrawing the sheath at the end of the case, particularly if a percutaneous approach has been used, it is critical that the blood pressure be monitored for 2 to 3 minutes because any acute drop is pathognomonic of an iliac rupture.

Retroperitoneal iliac exposure may be required if using cuff extenders and the device is not long enough to reach the location of the tear or if the femoral arteries are too small or calcified to use. If there has been pelvic trauma, using the side with the least hematoma is desirable. The common iliac can be accessed directly or a 10-mm silo graft is anastomosed end-to-side. If the pelvis is deep, to avoid a problem with angulation, the silo graft can be tunneled through the lower abdominal soft tissue or indeed through the femoral canal to the groin. Patients who have had prior aortoiliac grafts can be challenging because the iliacs are often imbedded in scar tissue. The ureter should always be mobilized anteriorly, avoiding dissection on both sides to prevent devascularization. In most cases the best that can be achieved is that enough dissection of the iliac limb of the graft allows application of a partial occlusion clamp or direct graft puncture. Having completed the procedure, whether anastomosing to graft or native vessel, the conduit is simply truncated and oversewn as a patch. In some circumstances it may be advisable to convert the conduit to an iliofemoral artery bypass. This allows a relatively easier access route for later percutaneous interventions should the need arise.

Some patients may already have an open abdomen, and in these cases direct infrarenal aortic access can be used [46]. This is not a good choice if there has been visceral spillage.

The procedure

Endovascular stent-grafting is an operative procedure, and should be performed in a room designed with this in mind, including sterile setup and laminar flow. It can be performed in a standard operating suite, using portable C-arm, but the image quality offered by multipurpose suites with fixed fluoroscopy units provides significantly better resolution. General anesthesia with a single-lumen endotracheal tube is sufficient. A right radial arterial line for blood pressure monitoring is optimal because the left subclavian may be covered or the left brachial artery needed for access. Depending on the angle needed best to visualize the arch, the arms may need to be elevated above the head or a bump placed under the left side. Before preparing, fluoroscopy should be performed to ensure that no tubes, lines, or boney structures obscure the field. The authors have found it helpful to place a 5- or 6-Fr catheter sheath and multimarker pigtail catheter through the femoral artery opposite to the side through which the device is deployed. This permits final angiographic marking with the nondeployed stent-graft in place. It also allows access for completion pelvic angiogram (although this can be done through the sheath) and access for a balloon occluder in the event of iliac rupture. Great care should be taken to avoid air or atheroemboli. In obese patients, or those with a weak pulse, ultrasound is very helpful in accessing the common femoral artery, and avoiding areas of significant plaque. After arterial access is established, 5000 units of heparin are administered, although it is possible to avoid heparinization if there is concern for bleeding complications [29]. A 5- or 6-Fr pigtail catheter is advanced over a floppy 3-J wire, and then the wire is exchanged for a stiffer wire (eg, an Amplatz or Lunderquist). The location of the rear of the wire should be marked on the table, so that any advancement or withdrawal can be detected. The delivery sheath is then advanced under constant fluoroscopic monitoring, usually in the anteroposterior view. Ideally, it should lie in the distal aorta. Once the device is in the approximate desired location, the image intensifier is rotated to the ideal angle, and angiography performed with respirations suspended. Usually 20 mL of contrast per second for 2 seconds is adequate. A road map can be obtained and the landmarks marked with a felt pen. At this point, the stent graft is deployed. The authors prefer to withdraw the pigtail used for angiogram below the stent before deployment. With most devices, deployment is rapid, and adenosine arrest is not needed. Hypertension should be avoided. Using cuff extenders, the authors prefer adenosine, at least for the first graft, to avoid distal displacement. When deploying cuffs, in general the authors have started distally, which they believe helps stabilize subsequent more proximal devices. Once the device is deployed, gentle ballooning, starting distally, is performed. When using multiple devices, the ballooning should proceed proximally, covering all areas of overlap. When deploying cuffs, the balloons do occlude the aorta, and even the trifascicular balloon when deployed across the curvature of the aorta can result in acute proximal hypertension and grab the stent graft. Ideally, in trauma cases, ballooning can be avoided altogether. If needed, rapid inflation and deflation with one third contrast and two thirds saline solution prevents significant hypertension. Vigorous overballooning should be avoided. The balloon should be withdrawn below the stent, maintaining wire access, and a completion angiogram performed. If there is a small endoleak or of there is a lip of the graft not being apposed to the inner curve of the aorta, repeat ballooning should be performed. If this fails to eradicate the issue, extending the graft with an additional module should be considered. Larger balloons can catch along the edge of the delivery sheath, but gently pulling the balloon and sheath beyond the aortoiliac junction usually allows balloon catheter to straighten out and be removed. The sheath is then gently withdrawn to as close to the inguinal ligament as possible (in the case of femoral access) and completion pelvic angiogram by the contralateral pigtail (or sheath if one was not placed) performed.

Follow-up

The protocols for follow-up are based on the various clinical trials designed predominantly to evaluate thoracic endografting for atherosclerotic aneurysms. Typical guidelines include CT angiography at 48 hours; discharge; 1, 6, and 12 months;

and then annually. These protocols are designed to detect graft collapse, migration, or persistent endoleak with aneurysmal growth. To a large extent, these guidelines were laid out because the cases involved patients with diseased landing zones with a potential for ongoing dilation of the aorta. Obvious concerns include following patients with renal insufficiency, and the burden of a large number of radiation exposures. Patients with renal insufficiency can be surveyed with intravascular ultrasound, transesophageal echocardiography, MR angiography, or even CT without contrast. The primary concern is whether or not there is pseudoaneurysm regression or growth. Simple chest radiography can detect stent deformation or migration. For aortic transection cases the authors tend to obtain a CT angiography at 48 hours, at 1 month, at 1 year, and then follow with chest radiographs. When obtaining a CT angiogram, it is important to make sure that the study is performed in a uniform manner: triphasic with unenhanced, enhanced, and delayed images. Indwelling pressure transducers, placed at the time of abdominal aortic endografting, continue to be studied and may, at least in select patients, provide a useful alternative to serial imaging [74].

The authors have not used antiplatelet agents for thoracic aortic stent grafting. They treat these like any other implant, however, and recommend antibiotic prophylaxis for any invasive procedure (eg, dental work).

Complications

Endoleak and endotension

Endoleak can be categorized as type I (leak around the proximal [A] or distal [B] ends of the graft); type II (leak from an artery feeding into the aneurysm sac); type III (leak between components); or type IV (failure of graft integrity). Typically, distal type I endoleak is rare in the trauma setting. These generally are found in patients with extensive atheromatous disease and dilated, short distal landing zones. Proximal type I endoleaks occur in approximately 5% of cases. Persistent type I endoleak is associated with a risk of late rupture [43]. The predominant mechanism in trauma patients is the combination of a short landing zone and lack of apposition along the inner curvature of the arch. Gentle ballooning should be tried first. If this is not sufficient, then extending proximally with another graft should follow [25,75]. Type I

leaks that are visualized only on delayed images immediately following deployment may resolve following heparin reversal. The authors assess these at 48 hours with a repeat CT angiogram. Blood pressure should be controlled with β-blockade during this period. Proximal type I endoleaks found on follow-up imaging usually can be managed by repeat interventions. Significant leaks seen at the time of implant, or at follow-up, that do not respond to further ballooning or extension should undergo operative repair. There have been attempts to coil embolize the pseudoaneurysm in the hope that thrombosis will ensue, but clinically and experimentally this does not seem to reduce the endotension and is associated with a risk of late rupture. Most type I endoleaks occur within 30 days, but occasionally can be found up to 2 years later, reinforcing the need for strict surveillance.

Type II endoleaks should be managed based on whether or not the left subclavian is the source. If it is, coil occlusion of the subclavian, carotid to subclavian bypass with proximal ligation, or carotid subclavian to carotid transposition should be performed. Left subclavian arterial causes of type II endoleak are less common in the trauma setting than the more typical atherosclerotic aneurysm case where there is circumferential dilation and the subclavian is more likely to feed into the aneurysm. Type II endoleaks believed to be secondary to patent bronchial or intercostal arteries are more problematic, but again are less problematic in the trauma setting because there are fewer branches in the proximal descending thoracic aorta. Some investigators believe that these are more benign than in the setting of abdominal endografting, and that in most cases they seal spontaneously [76]. Rarely, a branch vessel can be accessed and coiled using microcatheter techniques (Fig. 7).

Type III endoleaks represent a leak between endograft components, and are expected to be seen predominantly when cuff extenders are used, particularly if deployed along the curvature of the distal arch and proximal descending aorta. These are usually seen at the time of implant, and are managed by repeat ballooning or deploying another cuff across the site of the leak (Fig. 8).

Type IV endoleak has not been described to the authors' knowledge in the trauma population but implies a general failure of the graft material. Endotension refers to persistent pressure within an aneurysm or pseudoaneurysm without a documented endoleak. Clearly, if there is a source that can be defined it should be addressed. If no source

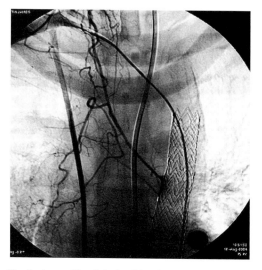

Fig. 7. A type II endoleak arising from an aberrant connection between a bronchial artery and the thyrocervical artery. This latter was selectively cannulized, the sac injected with biologic glue, and the feeding branch embolized.

is identified, but there is continued aneurysm growth, most surgeons opt for operative repair rather than re-endografting. There is debate about whether absence of regression without growth represents evidence of endotension. Regardless, this does not seem to be a concern in most trauma

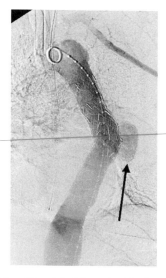

Fig. 8. A type III endoleak (*arrow*) arising between components of cuff extenders used to treat a chronic post-traumatic aneurysm. This was managed by deploying another cuff across the site of leak and reballooning.

patients, and the authors' own bias is that if the pseudoaneurysm is completely thrombosed following endografting, then routine follow-up is all that is required.

Stent graft collapse

This is a catastrophic complication that can occur immediately, or within the first 48 hours, but it has been seen up to 3 months postprocedure [77]. It is believed that this represents a combination of graft oversizing and a lack of apposition along the inner curve of the aorta. In young hyperdynamic aortas, with their degree of pliability, the force of the cardiac ejection that hits the underside of the graft causes collapse of the graft. This usually leads to immediate aortic occlusion and possibly rupture. If this occurs postimplant, the patient develops signs of acute coarctation, and the rapid onset of paralysis and renal failure can occur. This may not be immediately apparent if the patient is still on the ventilator and sedated. Prevention includes very accurate sizing, choosing a graft that approximates a 10% oversizing rather than 20%. It is also important to plan preoperatively and intraoperatively to avoid landing in the "no man's land" of the aorta. If the proximal portion of the graft is not apposed or at least close to the inner curve, particularly if there is only a short zone of apposition, perhaps less than 50%, then options include extending the graft proximally or repeat ballooning [77]. Uncovered bare metal stents deployed within the stent graft have also been used both acutely and when collapse occurs in a delayed fashion. There has been some concern that these bare stents may either erode over time through the graft fabric or create proximal aortic perforations [40]. There are not enough data to determine the real risk of this occurring, but theoretically a short bare stent conforms more closely to the aortic curvature than a bare proximal portion that is secured to an endograft and has reduced flexibility. Nationwide there have been numerous anecdotal reports of bare stent extenders being used for proximal partial or complete collapse with good short-term results. There is growing consensus that cuff extenders, which may be deployed sequentially and fit the curvature of the aorta better, may prove to perform better than longer thoracic stent grafts in patients with aortic diameters smaller than 24 mm.

If stent graft collapse occurs postoperatively, it can often be detected by plain chest radiography or by noncontrast CT. Immediate intervention is required. If complete collapse has occurred, explanting and operative repair is prudent, but ballooning and extending the device with a bare stent has been used with success [29]. Anectodotally, axillary-femoral-femoral bypass has been used as a temporizing measure, but ultimately the stent must be removed.

Stroke

Stroke remains a problem with thoracic endografting, occurring at a rate of 3% to 5% of cases. In the trauma population the incidence is lower, at 0% to 2% depending on the series [28]. Occlusion of a critical left vertebral artery is one cause. There are some data that aberrant vertebrals arising from the arch directly may be more likely to be a major source of posterior circulation, and in these cases the authors are more apt first to perform vertebral transfer. In older patients, arch thrombus is a concern for its embolic risk. Manipulation with the stiff wire across the arch can cause embolization. This has not been demonstrated in the trauma population to the authors' knowledge, but should it happen, theoretical options include immediate cerebral angiography and if there is a definitive lesion, intervention with catheter-based techniques. Finally, inadvertent guidewire advancement into carotid, or air embolism because of a loose connection, can result in cerebrovascular events. Whenever a catheter is proximal to the left subclavian artery, meticulous deairing of the catheter and equipment is mandatory. Wire position should be monitored and stabilized at all times. Never advance a catheter or wire blindly.

Embolization

Distal embolization is more of a concern in older patients with diffuse atheromata. Rarely, a traumatic injury can present with thrombus arising from the injury site (Fig. 9). In any patient where there is a recognized risk that wire or device manipulation might cause distal embolization, one should be prepared to perform distal angiography and to record distal pulses at the start and end of the procedure.

Bronchial obstruction

Grafts placed in the mid-descending aorta have rarely been associated with compression of the left main bronchus [78]. This may be detected on follow-up CT or chest radiograph, bronchoscopy for

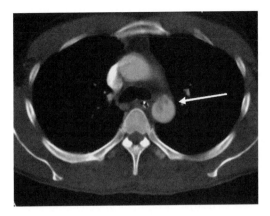

Fig. 9. An acute rupture presenting with thrombus at the site of injury. There is a risk that thrombus can be dislodged during wire manipulation, and the patient should be monitored postoperatively for evidence of visceral or peripheral changes.

other reasons, or clinically with new-onset asthma. The optimal management is open repair of the aorta and explanting the device when medically feasible. Bronchial stenting predisposes to the development of aortobronchial fistula.

Implant syndrome

Occasionally, patients experience persistent or new back pain, fever, malaise, or flulike syndrome following implantation. This has been reported more commonly with abdominal aortic endografting, but Rousseau and associates [6] found it in nearly one fifth of their series [79,80]. It is not clear whether or not the back pain is caused by residual endotension, inflammation secondary to the thrombosis in the excluded aorta, or a systemic inflammatory response to the graft. Repeat CT angiography is required to rule out a complication, but the presence of elevated erythrocyte sedimentation rate, with or without leukocytosis, and a normal CT suggest the diagnosis. Many patients also complain of various degrees of pleurisy. This condition is self-limited, usually resolving within 7 days, and can be treated with anti-inflammatory medications.

Dissection or rupture

Free rupture can occur at any time. Prevention is strict blood pressure control, particularly during periods of transfer or other procedures that might acutely elevate the heart rate or blood pressure. At the time of initial wire passage, great care should be given to watching the wire advance. If there is difficulty negotiating the aortic curvature or there is narrowing at the injury site, a directional catheter, such as a vertebral or hydrophilic catheter, can be invaluable.

There have been cases of delayed or immediate rupture after the graft has been deployed. Endografts that feature a bare metal proximal extension have been implicated in perforating the aortic wall [81]. Even covered grafts that do not have this feature have been implicated if there is poor apposition of the aortic wall with resultant motion against the wall. All three dedicated thoracic endografts discussed here have been implicated in acute or delayed perforation with or without dissection, at least anecdotally, in the nontrauma experience. Proper graft sizing is essential to facilitate good graft-aortic apposition.

Proximal dissection has also been documented. One mechanism is that during ballooning of the proximal cuff, the ends of the graft can create a dissection flap that rapidly progresses retrograde. To avoid this, initial ballooning should be as gentle as possible, just enough to document profiling of the balloon along the side of the graft. Ballooning should only be done within the graft.

Migration

If the proximal landing zone is not long enough, and the aneurysm itself is large, stents can migrate distally. This may be detected on routine chest radiograph, or may present with a new endoleak. In younger patients, as aortic growth occurs, an endograft may loose its fixation. If this should occur, options include both operative explanting and grafting, or proximal extension with another endograft. This is one of the reasons that lifelong surveillance is necessary.

Paralysis

The risk of paralysis with endografting in the trauma setting has not been seen in the recent series. This is presumably because in most cases only a short segment of the proximal descending aorta is covered. Based on experience acquired from treating atherosclerotic aneurysms, however, there may be uncommon circumstances (eg, treating a chronic posttraumatic aneurysm in an older patient) where there is increased risk. The major risk factors include covering more than 20 cm of aorta and prior abdominal aortic procedures. These risks are enhanced if the left subclavian must be covered, or if there is extensive iliac disease with hypogastric occlusion. In the elective setting, placement of a lumbar drain and allowing increased pressure after the endograft procedure can both reduce the risk of paralysis or, in as many as one third to one half of patients who do develop neurologic changes, reverse the spinal cord ischemia [82,83]. This is not a viable option in most acute trauma settings, but may be considered in delayed or elective settings.

Other long-term complications

Aortobronchial or aortofistula have been reported years after endografting [84]. Sayed and Thompson [20] reviewed 1518 cases reported in the literature of thoracic endografting (primarily for nontraumatic thoracic aneurismal disease) and found six cases (0.4%) of thoracic graft infection, paralleling the experience with abdominal grafts [85]. The primary risk factor was other intravascular sources of infection. Surgical management was associated with a 16% mortality compared with 36% with medical management alone. Any evidence of aneurysmal changes or persistent bacteremia should prompt consideration for surgical intervention.

Regulatory issues and consent implications

It is important to clarify that use of endovascular stent grafting for acute traumatic injuries is not approved by the Food and Drug Administration. When discussing the plan with patients or families, this should be made clear and documented. In particular, the lack of long-term follow-up should be discussed in the context of the long-term efficacy of the open repair, and a clear rational as to why an endovascular approach is preferred should be explained. It is useful to remember that these devices are engineered for a 10-year life span. The authors have no data about longer-term durability. It is also important to review the follow-up that is required, including the need for additional radiation exposure.

The pediatric and adolescent patient

Endovascular aortic stent grafts are not commonly used in pediatric and adolescent patients (Fig. 10) [86]. These patients usually have aortas that are too small for currently available devices that will likely grow, and the lack of long-term durability has greater significance in this population.

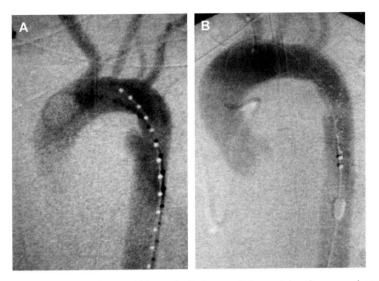

Fig. 10. (*A*) A traumatic injury in a 12-year-old boy who had severe intracranial, pulmonary, visceral, and pelvic injuries. The patient also has an aberrant origin of the left vertebral artery. Note the blurring of the image associated with an intraoperative imaging system, less clear than those obtained in a dedicated suite. (*B*) Post stent repair. At 4 years follow-up there have been no complications.

Future trends

Endograft technology is continuing to evolve, but perhaps even more significantly, experience and longer follow-up data are beginning to accrue. Branched grafts are beginning to be designed for both arch and abdominal visceral vessels. Specific for the trauma population, a variety of grafts that are shorter, precurved, and smaller are being developed, which allows more precise deployment and potentially reduced complication rates.

Summary

Endovascular repair of the traumatically injured thoracic aorta has emerged as an exceptionally promising modality that is typically quicker than open repair, with a reduced risk of paralysis. There are a specific set of anatomic criteria that need to be applied, which can be rapidly assessed by the CT angiogram. The enthusiasm for endovascular repair must be tempered by recognition of the complications and lack of long-term follow-up, particularly in younger patients. Surgeons who are skilled in open aortic repair must not only be involved, but should take on a leadership role during the planning, deployment, and follow-up of these patients. Familiarity with all of the available devices expands treatment options. As

more specific devices become available, and more follow-up is accrued, the role of endovascular stents will continue to grow.

References

[1] Parmley L, Mattingly T, Manion W, et al. Nonpenetrating traumatic injury of the aorta. Circulation 1958;17:1086–101.

[2] Mattox KL, Wall MJ Jr. Historical review of blunt injury to the thoracic aorta. Chest Surg Clin N Am 2000;10:167–82.

[3] Holmes J 3rd, Bloch RD, Hall RA, et al. Natural history of traumatic rupture of the thoracic aorta managed nonoperatively: a longitudinal analysis. Ann Thorac Surg 2002;73:1149–54.

[4] Pate JW, Gavant ML, Weiman DS, et al. Traumatic rupture of the aortic isthmus: program of selective management. World J Surg 1999;23:59–63.

[5] Kepros J, Angood P, Jaffe CC, et al. Aortic intimal injuries from blunt trauma: resolution profile in nonoperative management. J Trauma 2002;52:475–8.

[6] Rousseau H, Dambrin C, Marcheix B, et al. Acute traumatic aortic rupture: a comparison of surgical and stent-graft repair. J Thorac Cardiovasc Surg 2005;129:1050–5.

[7] Miller PR, Kortesis BG, McLaughlin CA III, et al. Complex blunt aortic injury or repair: beneficial effects of cardiopulmonary bypass use. Ann Surg 2003;237:877–83 [discussion: 883–4].

[8] Karmy-Jones R, Carter YM, Nathens A, et al. Impact of presenting physiology and associated injuries

on outcome following traumatic rupture of the thoracic aorta. Am Surg 2001;67:61–6.

[9] Forbes AD, Ashbaugh DG. Mechanical circulatory support during repair of thoracic aortic injuries improves morbidity and prevents spinal cord injury. Arch Surg 1994;129:494–7 [discussion: 497–8].

[10] Fabian TC, Richardson JD, Croce MA, et al. Prospective study of blunt aortic injury: Multicenter Trial of the American Association for the Surgery of Trauma. J Trauma 1997;42:374–80 [discussion: 380–3].

[11] Cook J, Salerno C, Krishnadasan B, et al. The effect of changing presentation and management on the outcome of blunt rupture of the thoracic aorta. J Thorac Cardiovasc Surg 2006;131:594–600.

[12] Arajarvi E, Santavirta S. Chest injuries sustained in severe traffic accidents by seatbelt wearers. J Trauma 1989;29:37–41.

[13] Kato N, Dake MD, Miller DC, et al. Traumatic thoracic aortic aneurysm: treatment with endovascular stent-grafts. Radiology 1997;205:657–62.

[14] Dake MD, Miller DC, Mitchell RS, et al. The first generation of endovascular stent-grafts for patients with aneurysms of the descending thoracic aorta. J Thorac Cardiovasc Surg 1998;116:689–703 [discussion: 703–4].

[15] Fujikawa T, Yukioka T, Ishimaru S, et al. Endovascular stent grafting for the treatment of blunt thoracic aortic injury. J Trauma 2001;50:223–9.

[16] Lawlor DK, Ott M, Forbes TL, et al. Endovascular management of traumatic thoracic aortic injuries. Can J Surg 2005;48:293–7.

[17] Lebl DR, Dicker RA, Spain DA, et al. Dramatic shift in the primary management of traumatic thoracic aortic rupture. Arch Surg 2006;141:177–80.

[18] Kuhne CA, Ruchholtz S, Voggenreiter G, et al. [Traumatic aortic injuries in severely injured patients]. Unfallchirurg 2005;108:279–87 [in German].

[19] Uzieblo M, Sanchez LA, Rubin BG, et al. Endovascular repair of traumatic descending thoracic aortic disruptions: should endovascular therapy become the gold standard? Vasc Endovascular Surg 2004; 38:331–7.

[20] Sayed S, Thompson MM. Endovascular repair of the descending thoracic aorta: evidence for the change in clinical practice. Vascular 2005;13:148–57.

[21] Wellons ED, Milner R, Solis M, et al. Stent-graft repair of traumatic thoracic aortic disruptions. J Vasc Surg 2004;40:1095–100.

[22] Andrassy J, Weidenhagen R, Meimarakis G, et al. Stent versus open surgery for acute and chronic traumatic injury of the thoracic aorta: a single-center experience. J Trauma 2006;60:765–71 [discussion: 771–2].

[23] Thompson CS, Rodriguez JA, Ramaiah VG, et al. Acute traumatic rupture of the thoracic aorta treated with endoluminal stent grafts. J Trauma 2002;52:1173–7.

[24] Orford VP, Atkinson NR, Thompson K, et al. Blunt traumatic aortic transection: the endovascular experience. Ann Thorac Surg 2003;75:106–12.

[25] Neuhauser B, Czermak B, Jaschke W, et al. Stent-graft repair for acute traumatic thoracic aortic rupture. Am Surg 2004;70:1039–44.

[26] Peterson BG, Matsumura JS, Morasch MD, et al. Percutaneous endovascular repair of blunt thoracic aortic transection. J Trauma 2005;59:1062–5.

[27] Marty-Ane CH, Berthet JP, Branchereau P, et al. Endovascular repair for acute traumatic rupture of the thoracic aorta. Ann Thorac Surg 2003;75: 1803–7.

[28] Dunham MB, Zygun D, Petrasek P, et al. Endovascular stent grafts for acute blunt aortic injury. J Trauma 2004;56:1173–8.

[29] Tehrani HY, Peterson BG, Katariya K, et al. Endovascular repair of thoracic aortic tears. Ann Thorac Surg 2006;82:873–7 [discussion: 877–8].

[30] Amabile P, Collart F, Gariboldi V, et al. Surgical versus endovascular treatment of traumatic thoracic aortic rupture. J Vasc Surg 2004;40:873–9.

[31] Fabian TC, Davis KA, Gavant ML, et al. Prospective study of blunt aortic injury: helical CT is diagnostic and antihypertensive therapy reduces rupture. Ann Surg 1998;227:666–76 [discussion: 676–7].

[32] Feliciano DV. Trauma to the aorta and major vessels. Chest Surg Clin N Am 1997;7:305–23.

[33] Maggisano R, Nathens A, Alexandrova NA, et al. Traumatic rupture of the thoracic aorta: should one always operate immediately? Ann Vasc Surg 1995;9:44–52.

[34] Mattison R, Hamilton IN Jr, Ciraulo DL, et al. Stent-graft repair of acute traumatic thoracic aortic transection with intentional occlusion of the left subclavian artery: case report. J Trauma 2001;51:326–8.

[35] Myburgh JA. Driving cerebral perfusion pressure with pressors: how, which, when? Crit Care Resusc 2005;7:200–5.

[36] Pace MC, Cicciarella G, Barbato E, et al. Severe traumatic brain injury: management and prognosis. Minerva Anestesiol 2006;72:235–42.

[37] Kinoshita K, Sakurai A, Utagawa A, et al. Importance of cerebral perfusion pressure management using cerebrospinal drainage in severe traumatic brain injury. Acta Neurochir Suppl 2006;96:37–9.

[38] Czosnyka M, Hutchinson PJ, Balestreri M, et al. Monitoring and interpretation of intracranial pressure after head injury. Acta Neurochir Suppl 2006; 96:114–8.

[39] Fisher RG, Oria RA, Mattox KL, et al. Conservative management of aortic lacerations due to blunt trauma. J Trauma 1990;30:1562–6.

[40] Malina M, Brunkwall J, Ivancev K, et al. Late aortic arch perforation by graft-anchoring stent: complication of endovascular thoracic aneurysm exclusion. J Endovasc Surg 1998;5:274–7.

[41] Borsa JJ, Hoffer EK, Karmy-Jones R, et al. Angiographic description of blunt traumatic injuries to

the thoracic aorta with specific relevance to endograft repair. J Endovasc Ther 2002;9(Suppl 2): II84–91.

[42] Wheatley GH III, Gurbuz AT, Rodriguez-Lopez JA, et al. Midterm outcome in 158 consecutive Gore TAG thoracic endoprostheses: single center experience. Ann Thorac Surg 2006;81:1570–7 [discussion: 1577].

[43] Fattori R, Nienaber CA, Rousseau H, et al. Results of endovascular repair of the thoracic aorta with the Talent Thoracic stent graft: the Talent Thoracic Retrospective Registry. J Thorac Cardiovasc Surg 2006; 132:332–9.

[44] Scheinert D, Krankenberg H, Schmidt A, et al. Endoluminal stent-graft placement for acute rupture of the descending thoracic aorta. Eur Heart J 2004; 25:694–700.

[45] Hoffer EK, Karmy-Jones R, Bloch RD, et al. Treatment of acute thoracic aortic injury with commercially available abdominal aortic stent-grafts. J Vasc Interv Radiol 2002;13:1037–41.

[46] Karmy-Jones R, Hoffer E, Meissner MH, et al. Endovascular stent grafts and aortic rupture: a case series. J Trauma 2003;55:805–10.

[47] Nagy K, Fabian T, Rodman G, et al. Guidelines for the diagnosis and management of blunt aortic injury: an EAST Practice Management Guidelines Work Group. J Trauma 2000;48:1128–43.

[48] Mattox KL. Red River anthology. J Trauma 1997; 42:353–68.

[49] Dyer DS, Moore EE, Ilke DN, et al. Thoracic aortic injury: how predictive is mechanism and is chest computed tomography a reliable screening tool? A prospective study of 1,561 patients. J Trauma 2000; 48:673–82 [discussion: 682–3].

[50] Miller PR, Moore PS, Mansell E, et al. External fixation or arteriogram in bleeding pelvic fracture: initial therapy guided by markers of arterial hemorrhage. J Trauma 2003;54:437–43.

[51] Cardarelli MG, McLaughlin JS, Downing SW, et al. Management of traumatic aortic rupture: a 30-year experience. Ann Surg 2002;236:465–9 [discussion: 469–70].

[52] Downing SW, Sperling JS, Mirvis SE, et al. Experience with spiral computed tomography as the sole diagnostic method for traumatic aortic rupture. Ann Thorac Surg 2001;72:495–501 [discussion: 501–2].

[53] Chen MY, Regan JD, D'Amore MJ, et al. Role of angiography in the detection of aortic branch vessel injury after blunt thoracic trauma. J Trauma 2001; 51:1166–71 [discussion: 1172].

[54] Karmy-Jones R, DuBose R, King S. Traumatic rupture of the innominate artery. Eur J Cardiothorac Surg 2003;23:782–7.

[55] Smith MD, Cassidy JM, Souther S, et al. Transesophageal echocardiography in the diagnosis of traumatic rupture of the aorta. N Engl J Med 1995; 332:356–62.

[56] Goarin JP, Cluzel P, Gosgnach M, et al. Evaluation of transesophageal echocardiography for diagnosis of traumatic aortic injury. Anesthesiology 2000;93: 1373–7.

[57] Fischer CH, Campos Filho O, Palma da Fonseca JH, et al. [Use of transesophageal echocardiography during implantation of aortic endoprosthesis (stent): initial experience]. Arq Bras Cardiol 2001; 77:1–8 [in Spanish].

[58] Cinnella G, Dambrosio M, Brienza N, et al. Transesophageal echocardiography for diagnosis of traumatic aortic injury: an appraisal of the evidence. J Trauma 2004;57:1246–55.

[59] Uflacker R, Horn J, Phillips G, et al. Intravascular sonography in the assessment of traumatic injury of the thoracic aorta. AJR Am J Roentgenol 1999; 173:665–70.

[60] Fishman JE. Imaging of blunt aortic and great vessel trauma. J Thorac Imaging 2000;15:97–103.

[61] Vignon P, Boncoeur MP, Francois B, et al. Comparison of multiplane transesophageal echocardiography and contrast-enhanced helical CT in the diagnosis of blunt traumatic cardiovascular injuries. Anesthesiology 2001;94:615–22 [discussion 5A].

[62] Fattori R, Napoli G, Lovato L, et al. Indications for, timing of, and results of catheter-based treatment of traumatic injury to the aorta. AJR Am J Roentgenol 2002;179:603–9.

[63] Gorich J, Asquan Y, Seifarth H, et al. Initial experience with intentional stent-graft coverage of the subclavian artery during endovascular thoracic aortic repairs. J Endovasc Ther 2002;9(Suppl 2): II39–43.

[64] Hoppe H, Hohenwalter EJ, Kaufman JA, et al. Percutaneous treatment of aberrant right subclavian artery aneurysm with use of the Amplatzer septal occluder. J Vasc Interv Radiol 2006;17:889–94.

[65] Peterson BG, Eskandari MK, Gleason TG, et al. Utility of left subclavian artery revascularization in association with endoluminal repair of acute and chronic thoracic aortic pathology. J Vasc Surg 2006;43:433–9.

[66] Rehders TC, Petzsch M, Ince H, et al. Intentional occlusion of the left subclavian artery during stent-graft implantation in the thoracic aorta: risk and relevance. J Endovasc Ther 2004;11:659–66.

[67] Appoo JJ, Moser WG, Fairman RM, et al. Thoracic aortic stent grafting: improving results with newer generation investigational devices. J Thorac Cardiovasc Surg 2006;131:1087–94.

[68] Morasch MD, Kibbe MR, Evans ME, et al. Percutaneous repair of abdominal aortic aneurysm. J Vasc Surg 2004;40:12–6.

[69] Eggebrecht H, von Birgelen C, Naber C, et al. Impact of gender on femoral access complications secondary to application of a collagen-based vascular closure device. J Invasive Cardiol 2004;16:247–50.

[70] Hoffer EK, Bloch RD. Percutaneous arterial closure devices. J Vasc Interv Radiol 2003;14:865–85.

[71] Castelli P, Caronno R, Piffaretti G, et al. Incidence of vascular injuries after use of the Angio-Seal closure device following endovascular procedures in a single center. World J Surg 2006;30:280–4.

[72] Biancari F, Ylonen K, Mosorin M, et al. Lower limb ischemic complications after the use of arterial puncture closure devices. Eur J Vasc Endovasc Surg 2006;32:217–25.

[73] Watelet J, Gallot JC, Thomas P, et al. Percutaneous repair of aortic aneurysms: a prospective study of suture-mediated closure devices. Eur J Vasc Endovasc Surg 2006;32:261–5.

[74] Ellozy SH, Carroccio A, Lookstein RA, et al. First experience in human beings with a permanently implantable intrasac pressure transducer for monitoring endovascular repair of abdominal aortic aneurysms. J Vasc Surg 2004;40:405–12.

[75] Orend KH, Scharrer-Pamler R, Kapfer X, et al. [Endoluminal stent-assisted management of acute traumatic aortic rupture]. Chirurg 2002;73:595–600 [in German].

[76] Mertens R, Valdes F, Kramer A, et al. [Endovascular treatment of descending thoracic aorta aneurysm]. Rev Med Chil 2003;131:617–22 [in Spanish].

[77] Idu MM, Reekers JA, Balm R, et al. Collapse of a stent-graft following treatment of a traumatic thoracic aortic rupture. J Endovasc Ther 2005; 12:503–7.

[78] Rousseau H, Soula P, Perreault P, et al. Delayed treatment of traumatic rupture of the thoracic aorta with endoluminal covered stent. Circulation 1999; 99:498–504.

[79] Gerasimidis T, Sfyroeras G, Trellopoulos G, et al. Impact of endograft material on the inflammatory response after elective endovascular abdominal aortic aneurysm repair. Angiology 2005;56:743–53.

[80] Galle C, De Maertelaer V, Motte S, et al. Early inflammatory response after elective abdominal aortic aneurysm repair: a comparison between endovascular procedure and conventional surgery. J Vasc Surg 2000;32:234–46.

[81] D'Ancona G, Bauset R, Normand JP, et al. Endovascular stent-graft repair of a complicated penetrating ulcer of the descending thoracic aorta: a word of caution. J Endovasc Ther 2003;10:928–31.

[82] Cheung AT, Pochettino A, McGarvey ML, et al. Strategies to manage paraplegia risk after endovascular stent repair of descending thoracic aortic aneurysms. Ann Thorac Surg 2005;80:1280–8 [discussion: 1288–9].

[83] Cheung AT, Weiss SJ, McGarvey ML, et al. Interventions for reversing delayed-onset postoperative paraplegia after thoracic aortic reconstruction. Ann Thorac Surg 2002;74:413–9 [discussion: 420–1].

[84] Eggebrecht H, Baumgart D, Radecke K, et al. Aortoesophageal fistula secondary to stent-graft repair of the thoracic aorta. J Endovasc Ther 2004;11: 161–7.

[85] Fiorani P, Speziale F, Calisti A, et al. Endovascular graft infection: preliminary results of an international enquiry. J Endovasc Ther 2003;10:919–27.

[86] Milas ZL, Milner R, Chaikoff E, et al. Endograft stenting in the adolescent population for traumatic aortic injuries. J Pediatr Surg 2006;41:e27–30.

ELSEVIER
SAUNDERS

Thorac Surg Clin 17 (2007) 129–135

THORACIC
SURGERY
CLINICS

Index

Note: Page numbers of article titles are in **boldface** type.

A

Abdominal esophageal leak
and diversion, 70, 71

Acute respiratory distress syndrome, 12–15, 57, 58

Airway injuries, 35–45
and bronchoscopy, 38, 39
and pneumothorax, 37, 38
and subcutaneous emphysema, 37, 39

Airway management
and tracheobronchial injuries, 39, 40

Airways
and thoracic trauma, 6

Aortic and arterial lacerations, 104, 105

Aortic aneurysm
chronic traumatic, 97, 98

Aortic injuries, 2, 6, 7, 95–105, 111
delayed surgical repair of, 100, 101, 111

Aortic trauma, 95–98
endovascular approach to, 109–125

ARDS. See *Acute respiratory distress syndrome.*

Aristotle
and thoracic trauma, 1

Atelectrauma, 12, 13

Atrial rupture, 90

Auto-PEEP
and ventilation, 15

B

BAI. See *Blunt aortic injury.*

BAL. See *Bronchoalveolar lavage.*

Ballistics
and thoracic trauma, 3

Barotrauma, 12, 66

Bi-level positive airway pressure
and ventilation, 13, 14

BiPAP. See *Bi-level positive airway pressure.*

Blast injuries
and flail chest, 25
and lung injuries, 57

Bleeding
and video-assisted thoracic surgery, 77

Blood vessels
trauma to, 2, 6, 7, 95–105, 111

Blunt aortic disruption. See *Blunt aortic injury,* 96, 97

Blunt aortic injury, 95–98
and associated injuries, 2
delayed surgical repair of, 100, 101
and falls, 95
incidence of, 95, 96
and motor vehicle accidents, 95, 96, 109
and osseous pinch, 97
pathology of, 96–98
and stretching, 96, 97
and sudden blood pressure elevation, 97
and water-hammer effect, 97

Blunt traumatic lung injuries, **57–61**

Boerhaave's tear, 69

Bromfield, William
and thoracic trauma, 1

Bronchial obstruction
and endovascular repair, 123

Bronchoalveolar lavage
and ventilator-assisted pneumonia, 17, 18

Bronchoscopy
and airway injuries, 38, 39

C

Cardiac trauma, **87–93**

Cardiac valve injury, 89

thoracic.theclinics.com

Esophageal injuries, 62–71
    and abdominal esophageal leak, 70, 71
    and blunt trauma, 66
    and caustic ingestion, 64–66
    and cervical esophageal leak, 69
    diagnosis of, 66–67
    and diagnostic imaging, 65
    and endoscopic perforation, 63, 64
    and foreign body ingestion, 64–66
    and gunshot wounds, 63
    and laboratory studies, 67
    and motor vehicle accidents, 66
    and noncontained perforations, 69, 70
    and penetrating trauma, 63
    and stab wounds, 63
    and swallow studies, 67
    and thoracic esophageal leak, 69, 70
    and thoracic trauma, 7
    and tracheobronchial trauma, 37
    treatment of, 67–71
    treatment-related, 63, 64

Esophageal stricture
    noncontained perforation after dilation of, 69,
        70

Esophageal trauma, **62–71**

Esophagus
    anatomy of, 62–64
    necrotic, 70, 71

Extra-anatomic air
    and thoracic trauma, 4

F

Falls
    and blunt aortic injury, 95
    and diaphragm injuries, 81
    and flail chest, 25
    and lung injuries, 57

FAST. See *Focused assessment with sonography for
    trauma.*

Flail chest, 5, 25–31
    and blast injuries, 25
    and continuous positive airway pressure, 28
    and epidural analgesia, 27
    and falls, 25
    initial evaluation of, 25–27
    and Injury Severity Score, 28
    and internal fixation, 28–30
    and mechanical ventilation, 28
    medical management of, 27
    and metal prostheses, 28–30

    outcome and prognosis of, 27, 28
    pathophysiology of, 25, 26
    and respiratory failure, 28
    and rib fracture, 25–31
    surgical management of, 28–30
    and thoracic paravertebral block, 27
    and ventilation, 27, 28

Focused assessment with sonography for trauma,
    48

Foreign bodies
    in the heart, 92
    ingestion of, 64–66

G

Galen
    and thoracic trauma, 1

Great vessel trauma, 6, 7, 95–105
    aortography for, 99
    chest radiography for, 98
    clinical presentation of, 98–100
    computed tomography for, 98, 99, 115, 116
    diagnostic studies for, 98–100
    magnetic resonance angiography for, 100
    management of, 100–105
    operative repair of, 100–102
    and spinal and lower body circulation, 102–104
    transesophageal echocardiography for, 99

Gunshot wounds
    and diaphragm injuries, 81
    and esophageal injuries, 63
    and heart injuries, 90
    and thoracic trauma, 3
    and tracheobronchial injuries, 36, 39

H

Hamman's sign, 7

Heart injuries, 87–92
    and atrial rupture, 90
    and blunt trauma, 87–89
    and cardiac valve injury, 89
    and commotio cordis, 87
    and coronary artery injuries, 89, 90
    and diagnostic imaging, 88, 89
    and falls, 87
    and foreign bodies, 92
    and gunshot wounds, 90
    and motor vehicle accidents, 87, 89
    and myocardial contusions, 87–89
    and penetrating trauma, 90–92
    and pericardial rupture, 87
    and stab wounds, 90
    and thoracic trauma, 8

Ventilator-associated lung injury
   pathophysiology of, 11–13

Ventilator-associated pneumonia, 17–19
   and bronchoalveolar lavage, 17, 18

Vesalius
   and aortic rupture, 95

Video-assisted thoracic surgery
   contraindications for, 77
   for hemothorax, 50, 52, 73–75
   for lung injuries, 60
   for management of bleeding, 77
   for pneumothorax, 75
   for posttraumatic empyema, 76

   rare applications of, 77
   in thoracic trauma, 73–78
   for traumatic diaphragm injuries, 75, 76

Video-assisted thoracic surgical applications in thoracic
   trauma, **73–79**

Volutrauma, 12

W

Water-hammer effect
   and blunt acute aortic disruption, 97

Moving?

Make sure your subscription moves with you!

To notify us of your new address, find your **Clinics Account Number** (located on your mailing label above your name), and contact customer service at:

E-mail: elspcs@elsevier.com

800-654-2452 (subscribers in the U.S. & Canada)
407-345-4000 (subscribers outside of the U.S. & Canada)

Fax number: 407-363-9661

Elsevier Periodicals Customer Service
6277 Sea Harbor Drive
Orlando, FL 32887-4800

*To ensure uninterrupted delivery of your subscription, please notify us at least 4 weeks in advance of move.